Cultural Competence in
Clinical Psychiatry

Cultural Competence in Clinical Psychiatry

Edited by

Wen-Shing Tseng, M.D.
Jon Streltzer, M.D.

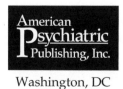

American Psychiatric Publishing, Inc.

Washington, DC
London, England

Note: The authors have worked to ensure that all information in this book is accurate at the time of publication and consistent with general psychiatric and medical standards, and that information concerning drug dosages, schedules, and routes of administration is accurate at the time of publication and consistent with standards set by the U.S. Food and Drug Administration and the general medical community. As medical research and practice continue to advance, however, therapeutic standards may change. Moreover, specific situations may require a specific therapeutic response not included in this book. For these reasons and because human and mechanical errors sometimes occur, we recommend that readers follow the advice of physicians directly involved in their care or the care of a member of their family.

Copyright © 2004 American Psychiatric Publishing, Inc.
ALL RIGHTS RESERVED

Manufactured in the United States of America on acid-free paper
08 07 06 05 04   5 4 3 2 1
First Edition

Typeset in Adobe's Palatino and ITC Highlander Book

American Psychiatric Publishing, Inc.
1000 Wilson Boulevard
Arlington, VA 22209-3901
www.appi.org

Library of Congress Cataloging-in-Publication Data
Cultural competence in clinical psychiatry/edited by Wen-Shing Tseng, Jon Streltzer.
    p. ; cm.
Includes bibliographical references and index.
ISBN 1-58562-125-0 (alk. paper)
    1. Cultural psychiatry. I. Tseng,Wen-Shing, 1935– II. Streltzer, Jon.
[DNLM: 1. Psychiatry--methods. 2. Clinical Competence. 3. Cross-Cultural Comparison. 4. Professional-Patient Relations. WM 100 C9675 2004]
RC455.4.E8C799 2004
616.89--dc22   2004046338

British Library Cataloguing in Publication Data
A CIP record is available from the British Library.

Contents

Case Vignettes

Contributors

Iqbal Ahmed, M.D.
Professor and Vice Chair, Department of Psychiatry; Program Director of General Psychiatric Training Program and Geriatric Psychiatric Program, University of Hawaii School of Medicine, Honolulu, Hawaii

Todd S. Elwyn, M.D., J. D.
Fellow, Forensic Psychiatry, and Clinical Teaching Assistant, University of Hawaii School of Medicine, Honolulu, Hawaii; Laughlin Fellow (2003) and Group for the Advancement of Psychiatry Fellow (2003–2004)

S. Peter Kim, M.D., Ph.D., M.B.A.
Professor of Psychiatry, Child-Adolescent Psychiatry Division, Department of Psychiatry, University of Hawaii School of Medicine, Honolulu, Hawaii

J. David Kinzie, M.D.
Professor of Psychiatry, School of Medicine, Oregon Health Sciences University; Founder, Indochinese Psychiatry Program, Portland, Oregon

Louise Lettich, M.D.
At the time of writing of this chapter, Dr. Lettich was Associate Professor of Psychiatry, University of Hawaii School of Medicine, and Director, Psychiatry Emergency Education Program, Honolulu, Hawaii. She is now in private practice in Massachusetts.

Paul K. Leung, M.D.
Associate Professor of Psychiatry and Director of Clinical Services, and Director, Intercultural Psychiatric Program, School of Medicine, Oregon Health Sciences University, Portland, Oregon

Cultural Competence in Clinical Psychiatry

Keh-Ming Lin, M.D., M.P.H.
Professor of Psychiatry, University of California at Los Angeles; Director, Research Center on the Psychobiology of Ethnicity, Harbor-UCLA Research and Education Institute, Los Angeles, California; Director, Division of Mental Health and Substance Abuse Research, National Health Research Institutes, Taiwan, R.O.C.

Francis G. Lu, M.D.
Professor of Clinical Psychiatry, University of California, San Francisco; Director, Cultural Competence and Diversity Program, Department of Psychiatry, San Francisco General Hospital, San Francisco, California

Daryl Matthews, M.D.
Professor of Psychiatry and Director, Forensic Psychiatry Program, University of Hawaii School of Medicine, Honolulu, Hawaii

Jon Streltzer, M.D.
Professor of Psychiatry and Director, Queen Emma Pain Clinic, University of Hawaii School of Medicine, Honolulu, Hawaii; Secretary, International College of Psychosomatic Medicine

Junji Takeshita, M.D.
Associate Professor of Psychiatry and Assistant Program Director, Geriatric Psychiatry Residency Program, University of Hawaii School of Medicine, Honolulu, Hawaii

Wen-Shing Tseng, M.D.
Professor of Psychiatry, University of Hawaii School of Medicine, Honolulu, Hawaii; Honorable Advisor, Transcultural Psychiatric Section of World Psychiatric Association

Joseph Westermeyer, M.D., M.P.H., Ph.D.
Professor of Psychiatry and Adjunct Professor of Anthropology, University of Minnesota; Chief of Psychiatry and Director of Mental Health Services, Veterans Affairs Medical Center, Minneapolis, Minnesota

Preface

That culture significantly influences the practice of medicine and psychiatry is undisputed. In the past, cultural psychiatry has typically been approached by examining populations of different ethnic groups, particularly minority groups. In this book, however, we take an entirely new approach: the examination of cultural issues as applied to the practice of various subfields of psychiatry. No book has yet met this need in a succinct, practical format.

We have previously edited two books that applied the principles of cultural psychiatry to clinical areas rather than specific ethnic groups. The first focused on assessment of psychopathology (Tseng and Streltzer 1997), and the second focused on psychotherapy (Tseng and Streltzer 2001). This book extends the direction of cultural psychiatry by addressing its application to various specialty areas within psychiatric practice. Our primary intention with this book is to foster cultural competence in specific services that will allow effective treatment of patients from any ethnic group.

As a whole, the book addresses theoretical and conceptual issues, but with emphasis on clinical applications. An introductory chapter presents general issues associated with cultural competence in assessing and treating patients. Particular issues relevant to specific services or specialties are covered in detail in the subsequent chapters. These include inpatient, outpatient, consultation-liaison and pain management, and emergency psychiatry. Other specialty areas include child and adolescent, geriatric, addiction, and forensic psychiatry. Chapters on psychopharmacology and psychotherapy cover these treatment modalities common to many of the subfields of psychiatry. Each chapter includes numerous case vignettes with discussion to provide concrete examples for the reader.

The book has been carefully edited for uniformity and integration. It is designed to serve as a practical guide that will be useful in meeting the new requirements for cultural competence in clinical work. The book will be useful for psychiatrists, psychologists, residents in training, and related mental health workers and students.

Wen-Shing Tseng, M.D.
Jon Streltzer, M.D.

References

Tseng WS, Streltzer J: Culture and Psychopathology: A Guide to Clinical Assessment. New York, Brunner/Mazel, 1997

Tseng WS, Streltzer J: Culture and Psychotherapy: A Guide to Clinical Practice. Washington, DC, American Psychiatric Press, 2001

1

Introduction

Culture and Psychiatry

Wen-Shing Tseng, M.D.
Jon Streltzer, M.D.

Culture and Its Influence on Medical Practice

What Is Culture?

The word *culture* refers to the unique behavior patterns and lifestyle shared by a group of people that distinguish it from other groups. A culture is characterized by a set of views, beliefs, values, and attitudes. Culture is manifested in the core of behavior and the various ways in which life is regulated, such as rituals, customs, etiquette, taboos, and laws. It is reflected in such things as common sayings, legends, drama, art, philosophical thought, and religions. Culture shapes people's behavior, but at the same time it is molded by the ideas and behavior of the members of the culture. Thus, culture and people influence each other reciprocally and interactionally. Culture is generally recognized in social or institutional patterns, and it affects specific behaviors and reactions of the individual. The individual may be aware of these influences or the influences may be operating at a subconscious level (Tseng 2001, p. 26).

Culture and Medical Practice

In the medical setting, three types of culture are present: the culture of the patient, the culture of the physician, and the medical culture in which the clinical work is practiced. An appropriate understanding of these three cultural dimensions is essential to the comprehension and performance of culturally competent clinical work.

The Culture of the Patient

In addition to individual factors—such as level of education, medical knowledge, and personal life experiences—culture will contribute to the patient's understanding of illness, perception and presentation of symptoms and problems, and reaction and adjustment to illness. The patient's expectations of the physician, motivation for treatment, and compliance with treatment recommendations are also influenced by culture.

The Culture of the Physician

Superimposed on individual style, personal belief, and professional knowledge, the culture of the physician will shape the pattern of inter-action and communication with the patient. For example, a physician might have cultural biases and expectations about the behavior and needs of a patient of a particular gender, sexual orientation, race, or eth-nicity; about a specific disease (such as acquired immune deficiency syndrome [AIDS] or alcohol abuse); or about a certain procedure (such as abortion). The culture of the physician explicitly or implicitly affects his or her attitude toward the patient, understanding of the patient's problems, and approach to caring for the patient.

The Medical Culture

Medical culture includes traditions, regulations, customs, and attitudes that have developed within the medical service setting beyond medical knowledge and theory. The practice of general psychiatry is strongly embedded in the medical culture that has developed within the medical system. Most physicians and medical staff members have become ac-customed to living within this invisible cultural system and may be un-aware of its influence on their practice. It often takes outsiders to recognize the existence of medical cultures, which may differ among specialties (such as surgery and psychiatry) but share common issues.

Examining medicine practiced in America, anthropologist H.F. Stein (1993) pointed out that for the American doctor, being in control is very important. The physician's dominant values are individualism (the doctor's ability to do the work himself), mastery over nature (capa-bility to cure the disease), and future orientation (being focused on the patient's eventual cure). Actively intervening, aggressively treating, controlling, and fixing the patient are acceptable attitudes for the clinician; these attitudes strongly reflect American value systems, which might not necessarily be shared in other cultures.

Whether the physician and nurse work together as egalitarian team members or in a distinct hierarchical order depends on the medical culture, which in turn reflects the culture of the society. How nurses and other medical staff members regard physicians varies in different cultural settings. For instance, in Japan, reflecting Japanese attitudes toward authority and male figures, male physicians are highly respected by medical staff and patients. Female nurses are accustomed to bowing to physicians and following orders obediently. In contrast, in America, the status of nurses is relatively high, and they often take charge in ward situations.

In medical practice it is believed that there should be a "diagnosis" for each patient. Without a diagnostic label on a patient's chart, the practice of medicine is not considered complete, and there can be no treatment. In addition, patients feel uncomfortable if they are not given a diagnosis and no medication is prescribed.

In psychiatry there are certain rules that patients and their families are asked to follow. Psychotherapy patients are supposed to visit their psychiatrists weekly, typically for 1 hour each session. This is based on the convenience of the therapist in an era of technical development and reflects the spirit of industrialized societies. In many parts of the world the concept of visiting a clinic for a scheduled appointment does not apply, reflecting the realities of societies where there are no private cars or public telephones. Patients drop in whenever it is convenient for them and when they feel like it. It is only when they practice in such settings that psychiatrists realize there is no point in trying to force their established medical expectations and culture on these patients.

Elements of Clinical Cultural Competence

To be clinically competent, every clinician needs to be culturally competent. Clinicians typically work in multiethnic, multicultural societies, providing care for patients of diverse backgrounds. The presence of diverse populations in a society creates the need for training in cultural psychiatry. Even when the cultural background of the patient is not significantly different from that of the clinician, it is inevitable that some differences will exist. Therefore, virtually all clinical practice can be considered to be transcultural (Comas-Díaz 1988).

Clinical cultural competence requires the attainment of several qualities (Foulks 1980; Lu et al. 1995; Moffic et al. 1988; Tseng and Streltzer 2001; Westermeyer 1989; Yutrzenka 1995). They include cultural sensitivity; cultural knowledge; cultural empathy; flexible, culturally relevant doctor-patient relations and interaction; and cultural guidance (the ability to use these qualities therapeutically) (Tseng 2001, 2003). These elements are elaborated in the following sections of this chapter.

Cultural Sensitivity

Cultural sensitivity refers to a recognition of the diversity of viewpoints, attitudes, and lifestyles among human beings. It includes the recognition that groups of people may tend to experience different types of stress in living and to utilize relatively distinctive coping patterns. Beyond being aware of these factors, the clinician needs to appreciate them without bias, prejudice, or stereotyping. Such appreciation requires a willingness to explore these areas and to learn from patients and their families about their beliefs, attitudes, value systems, and ways of dealing with problems. It is not only sensitive perception but also a desire to learn about others' lifestyles, rather than being trapped in one's own subjective perception and interpretation of their behavior.

Cultural Knowledge

In developing sensitivity it is helpful to have a certain base of cultural knowledge about humankind as a whole with which to put the particular patient and family into perspective. This is not to say that the clinician needs an anthropologist's knowledge of the subtleties and varieties of extant cultural systems. However, it is desirable to have some basic anthropological knowledge about how human beings vary in their habits, customs, beliefs, value systems, and especially illness behavior. This basic knowledge should be extended with regard to the cultural systems of patients, so that culturally relevant assessment and care can be delivered. Reading books and other literature is one way to obtain such cultural information. Consulting with medical anthropologists on general issues or with experts on a particular cultural system is another approach. When such material or consultation is not readily available, the patient and the family, or friends of the same ethnic-cultural background, may be used as resources. Of course, careful judgment is needed to determine the accuracy and relevance of the information obtained.

Cultural Empathy

An intellectual understanding about a patient's culture is often not sufficient for effective treatment. There is another quality needed: the ability to feel and understand, on an emotional level, the patient's own cultural perspective. The ability to participate in the emotional experience of the patient, known as cultural empathy (Pinderhughes 1984), is important to the quality of therapy.

Culturally Relevant Relations and Interactions

The interaction between the therapist and the patient involves the cultural background of both the patient and the therapist and the setting in which the therapy takes place. These influence not only the nature of the relationship between the therapist and the patient—in terms of role, status, and level of intimacy—but also issues of interaction, including communication, understanding, and giving and receiving between the therapist and patient. In particular, it is always necessary to consider the proper relation between an authoritative and a subservient figure and persons of different genders, and whether the setting is a professional or a social occasion or an accidental encounter. Such cultural knowledge will enhance clinical judgment, leading to a proper therapist-patient relationship that is culturally relevant and therapeutic.

The ability to detect, comprehend, and manage ethnic- or race-related transference and countertransference is also needed in dealing with patients of distinctly different ethnic or racial backgrounds. This is particularly true when problematic relationships have existed between the ethnic or racial groups of which the patient and therapist are members. For instance, the patient may be a member of a minority or majority group and the therapist the opposite. There may be a history of discrimination and an imbalance of power between these two groups. This interacts with the unequal roles of doctor and patient. The willingness of the therapist to give careful consideration to these issues, in order to properly manage and make appropriate adjustments to therapy, is important for cultural competence.

Cultural Guidance

Specific treatment models for particular ethnic groups are unlikely to be useful in clinical practice. There are so many kinds of problems within any given ethnic group that different therapeutic approaches must be applied accordingly. However, a certain general approach might be better suited to a specific ethnic group because of varying ways to relate to a doctor, cope with mental problems, and understand the role of psychiatric services.

To formulate the most effective intervention for patients in dealing with their problems, the clinician should assess the extent to which and the ways in which the patient's problems are related to cultural factors. Sometimes, direct advice should be given to challenge or adjust culturally determined norms, values, and goals so that the patient can cope with problems and resolve conflicts. Culturally sanctioned coping mechanisms may need to be reinforced or, if they are ineffective, to be confronted. Alternatives to culturally defined solutions may need to be proposed. To find relevant and optimal solutions, not only clinical judgment but also cultural insight and wisdom are sometimes required (Tseng and Streltzer 2001).

When the patient and therapist have different cultural backgrounds, therapy involves the interaction of two value systems. Thus, therapeutic interaction provides opportunities for exposure, exchange, and the incorporation of differing cultural elements between therapist and patient (Tseng and Hsu 1979). Cultural insight into the therapist's own beliefs and value system allows regulation of this core interaction and the overall therapeutic process in a competent manner.

Society, Culture, and Psychiatric Care: A General View

The practice of psychiatry occurs within a general context that includes the society, the cultures within it, and the medical system itself. Recognizing the social and cultural perspectives in which psychiatric service is delivered will present the clinician with more flexible therapeutic options.

Impact of Culture on Psychiatric Practice

Folk Concepts and Stigma of Mental Disorders

Even though modern psychiatry has made significant progress in its scientific understanding of the nature of psychiatric disorders, many people still believe various folk concepts about mental illness. Loss of soul, intrusion of illness objects, the wrongdoing of ancestors, deficiency of vitality, and an imbalance of yin and yang are some examples of folk interpretations of mental illness (Tseng 2001). An individual holding these beliefs might resist taking psychotropic medications. Such a patient may want to perform religious rituals to regain his or her "lost soul" or may want to eat certain foods to correct "an imbalance of yin and yang." Talking therapy is not considered to be effective for removing "an intruding ill spirit" or for correcting "deficient vitality."

Although increased knowledge and improvements in clinical care are changing peoples' attitudes toward mental disorders, there are still broad cultural differences in these attitudes. For instance, in Arab societies and in India, the mentally ill are respected and tolerated because of the historical notion that divine messages are sent through them. In contrast, in many societies, there is a general fear of and a strong stigma attached to "insane" people. These negative views of mental disorders obstruct the practice of psychiatric care.

Ethnicity, Minority, and Racism

Members of minority groups are often subjected to less favorable medical care, and psychiatric care and treatment are less likely to be available to them (Well et al. 1987). In general, this is the result of misperceptions and prejudice on the part of psychiatrists and, among patients, misconceptions and lack of knowledge about mental disorders and their treatments.

Concern about the effects of racism on psychiatric practice has been expressed since the 1970s in North America (Sabshin et al. 1970; Siegel 1974) and later in Western Europe (Burke 1984; Littlewood 1992). Minory patients tend to be given more severe clinical diagnoses. Misperceptions and miscommunication between doctor and patient occur because of patients' unfamiliarity with clinical settings and psychiatrists' unfamiliarity with symptom manifestation patterns and biased attitudes toward patients of certain ethnic or racial backgrounds. Mistrust on both sides interferes with the therapeutic relationship (Neki et al. 1985).

Patients who are members of minority groups tend to have fewer sessions and to drop out of treatment more frequently. They are more likely to receive biological or somatic treatments rather than psychotherapy. There is a risk that clinical care will be colored by subtle unfairness if not explicit discrimination (Kaplan and Busner 1992). Therefore, sensitive attention to race and minority status is critical to a therapeutic relationship (Collins et al. 1992; Griffith 1977).

Impact of the Social-Medical System

Number and Geographical Distribution of Psychiatrists

In different societies around the world, the number of psychiatrists available in a community varies tremendously, directly influencing the quality of psychiatric care (Tseng et al. 2001). In many developed societies there is a heavy concentration of psychiatrists in urban settings and a severe shortage in rural areas, even though the total number of psychiatrists in the society is relatively high. In many developing societies psychiatrists are very few in number and they focus mainly on those with severe mental illness.

Medical Insurance and Payment

Another factor that influences the mode of clinical practice is the extent to which psychiatric treatment is covered by medical insurance and whether the payment system is public or private. The payment system reflects the value placed by the society on the types of treatments available. For instance, in societies where talking therapy is not highly valued, it is difficult to charge patients very much for the service. This discourages psychiatrists from learning and performing this time-consuming therapy. In contrast, traditional medical habits and concepts deem it reasonable to charge for prescribing medications. Indirectly, this encourages drug-oriented treatment. Laboratory examinations using sophisticated scientific instruments usually qualify for high fees. This naturally leads to the performance of many unnecessary laboratory examinations such as brain scans or electroencephalograms for patients with psychological problems, who may not need these expensive examinations. Thus, payment systems, more than medical need, could shape the pattern of service delivery.

Legal and Ethical Aspects

Human Rights and Psychiatric Treatment

Certain issues of practice—such as involuntary hospitalization, the use of physical restraints, and involuntary administration of medications—are dealt with differently in various societies, and these differences may reflect basic attitudes and concepts about human rights. Thus cultural factors shape the way treatment is provided to patients with mental disorders.

Ethical Concerns

It is assumed that ethics apply absolutely and universally in medical practice. All physicians must keep the patients' best interests in mind in the course of care and, as much as possible, do them no harm. However, in cross-cultural applications this assumption may be arguable. Variations in ethics are observed from a cultural point of view and from international perspectives (Okasha et al. 2000). For instance, is it ethical for a physician to suggest sterilization for psychotic or mentally retarded patients? Is it ethical to treat homosexual persons as patients with a disorder?

In apartheid-era South Africa, when there was widespread political conflict between races, Steere and Dowdall (1990) pointed out that a set of ethical guidelines was likely to be plagued by recurrent dilemmas. A comparison of psychological ethics codes of 24 countries was made by Leach and Harbin (1997). They reported that Canada's code of ethics was the most similar to that of the American Psychological Association in the United States and that China's was the most dissimilar, demonstrating a relationship between professional ethical codes and cultural values.

Cultural Considerations in Clinical Practice

Cultural Differences in Therapist-Patient Relationships

Interpersonal relations are closely defined and regulated by social etiquette and cultural norms. This is particularly true for attitudes toward authority, which encompass the physician-patient relationship. In the United States, the predominant form of physician-patient relationship is egalitarian, based on a contractual agreement between the two and heavily influenced by an ideological emphasis on individualism, autonomy, and consumerism. In contrast, in many Asian cultures, the relationship is modeled after the ideal hierarchical relationship. The physician is seen as an authority figure who is clearly endowed with knowledge and experience. The ideal doctor should have great virtue and should be concerned, caring, and conscientiously responsible for the patient's welfare. In return, the patient must show respect and deference to the physician's authority and suggestions (Nilchaikovit et al. 1993).

Ethnic/Racial Transference and Countertransference

Ethnic or racial transference is a situation in which a patient develops a certain relationship, feeling, or attitude toward the therapist because of the therapist's ethnic or racial background. Ethnic or racial countertransference is the reverse phenomenon, in which a therapist's feelings and interventions are influenced by the patient's ethnic or racial background. Similar to personal transference or countertransference, ethnic or racial transference or countertransference can be positive or negative and can severely influence the process of therapy. It is therefore critical to recognize when treating the patient.

Ethnocultural transference may be manifested as denial of ethnicity and culture; mistrust, suspicion, and hostility; ambivalence toward the therapist; or overcompliance and friendliness (Comas-Díaz and Jacobsen 1991). Likewise, countertransference may be manifested as denial of ethnocultural differences; excessive curiosity about the patient's ethnocultural background; and excessive feelings of guilt, anger, or ambivalence toward the patient.

The possible negative impact of racism on psychiatric practice has attracted a great deal of attention (Carter 1995). In extreme circumstances psychotherapy can be quite difficult (Bizi-Nathaniel et al. 1991; Lambley and Cooper 1975), particularly when negative or even hostile relations preexist between the two racial groups concerned.

Being open with patients at an early stage of therapy about the possible effects of race and ethnic differences on therapy is encouraged as a way to minimize the ill effects associated with negative interracial relations (Brantley 1983).

Therapist-Patient Matching

Although the matching of therapist and patient by ethnicity, race, or cultural background sounds reasonable and desirable, it is not a simple matter. Such matching may not only be impractical, but clinically it does not necessarily guarantee success. Successful therapy relies on professional competence reflected in knowledge and experience. It also depends on the therapist's personal ability to establish a positive relationship with and show empathy toward the patient. In other words, although the matching of ethnic or cultural background might be beneficial, clinical competence could be more effective in bringing about desirable therapeutic outcomes. In addition, therapists with the same ethnic or racial backgrounds as their patients may sometimes be at a disadvantage. This can occur, for example, if the patient does not want to reveal his or her personal background to a therapist with the same background for fear of being judged harshly, or if the therapist does not offer a proper figure for ethnic identification.

Language

Languages vary greatly in their grammatical and communication patterns. For instance, differences in gender among subjects are noted in some languages (such as English, Russian, French, and Spanish) but not in others (such as Japanese and Chinese). This is related to the basic structure of the language, but it could also reflect the perceptions and conceptions of the people who use it. For instance, the vocabulary and grammar of the Japanese, with their hierarchical orientation, changes depending on the person to whom they are speaking.

The richness of variations and differentiations of certain words often indicates the level of concern for the subject in the culture. For instance, Westerners use different words to describe various kinds of wine or liquor, whereas the Chinese have only one inclusive word, "wine." In contrast, the Chinese use several different terms to address uncles or aunts, distinguishing paternal from maternal relatives and distinguishing hierarchically by age.

Meanings in Cultural Context

In psychiatric practice, it is important to grasp meanings expressed explicitly, tacitly, or in a symbolic way. Cultural idioms may invoke subtle or symbolic meanings of words. For instance, if someone says, "My house is far away," it might mean that you are not welcome to visit it. If someone asks whether you have already eaten, it might not mean the person is concerned about your eating or interested in offering you a meal, it may simply be a social greeting, like asking "How are you?" Even when a patient reveals a wish to kill himself, it should not necessarily be taken literally but requires a clinical judgment about the patient, his psychopathology, and the possible motivation for such a revelation. In addition, a cultural judgment is needed: an understanding of the general custom among people in the patient's culture of revealing a wish to end their lives, its common implication, and the possible message that the person wants to communicate. For example, if a Muslim person, whose faith forbids self-killing, expresses the wish that God would "take back" his life, the person may be indicating that he has suicidal thoughts, which must be taken seriously.

Culture-Shaped Communication Patterns

Beyond the words and language used for communication, cultural factors influence how a person communicates with others, both verbally and nonverbally, which has an impact on the clinical setting. It is well known that the Japanese tend to respond by saying, "Hai! Hai!" when they are being spoken to. Although *hai* in Japanese literally means "yes," it does not mean that the person is responding affirmatively to whatever is said. It simply indicates that he is listening to what is being said, even though he might disagree with it. In a similar way, a Filipino patient who keeps saying "Yes, doctor!" is not agreeing with the physician's instructions but is simply indicating respect for an authoritative figure with whom it is not proper to disagree (see "Case 4: A Quiet Man With High Blood Pressure," in Chapter 5, Culture and Consultation-Liaison Psychiatry).

Styles of Problem Presentation

A patient might make a somatic complaint not because she actually has a somatic problem but simply because it is a culture-patterned behavior to initially present somatic problems to a physician, or even to a psychiatrist. Sensitive probing, however, often reveals the more important emotional problems (Tseng 1975). In contrast, a patient might present a psychologized complaint—such as how much he hates his father or a trauma he encountered in his early childhood—at his first session with the therapist, as if he were very psychologically minded and aware of his psychological problems. However, as the therapy goes on, it might be shown that the patient learned to present such "psychoanalytical" material from the mass media or from his friends, whereas he actually knows nothing about his own psychological problems.

Disclosure of Personally Sensitive Information or Taboo Subjects

In general, a therapist would like to have the patient disclose as much personal information as possible so that a proper, in-depth understanding of the patient can be achieved. There are many cultural variations, however, regarding how much internal information a person should reveal to an outsider and what issues are taboo. For example, in many cultures (including Asian cultures) it is taboo to discuss imminent death from a terminal disease. In such a circumstance, breaking the social taboo and helping the person face reality and prepare for the end of life has to be done delicately and subtly, rather than discussing the subject openly and liberally. Otherwise, the patient might conclude that the therapist wishes him to die soon.

Confidentiality

Closely related to revealing private matters is how confidentiality is conceived and practiced in various cultural settings. If, in the patient's social setting, the rights of the individual are more or less emphasized and personal boundaries are relatively well established, confidentiality is understood and expected in the clinical situation. However, in a society where the group (or family) is emphasized and individual autonomy has less value, the patient or the family might assume that the therapist will share information, an assumption that could greatly complicate treatment.

Communication Through an Interpreter

When the therapist and the patient do not share the same language they need to rely on interpreters for communication. Selecting a proper interpreter and utilizing the interpreter for the goal of communication is a clinical skill and art (Kinzie 1985; Marcos 1979; Paniagua 1998). In general, it is desirable to have an interpreter who has knowledge and experience in mental health work. The interpreter needs orientation, and perhaps training, for the work to be done.

There may be problems in translating properly, relevantly, and meaningfully for clinical purposes. Deletion or omission of information, distortion of meaning, and exaggeration or addition of information are some of the problems that might be encountered with interpretation (Lee 1997). It has been reported that even when medically trained bilingual nurses were used as interpreters in medical settings, many serious miscommunication problems still occurred that affected either the physician's understanding of the symptoms or the credibility of the patient's concerns. Among the many factors that resulted in misunderstandings were the following: 1) physicians resisted reconceptualizing the problem when contradictory information was mentioned; 2) nurses (acting as interpreters) provided information congruent with clinical expectations but not congruent with the patient's comments; 3) nurses slanted the interpretation, reflecting unfavorably on the patients and undermining their credibility; and 4) patients explained their symptoms by using cultural metaphors that were not compatible with modern clinical nosology (Elderkin-Thompson et al. 2001).

There are several different ways to use an interpreter. Word-for-word translation is needed in areas that are delicate and significant; summary translation, in areas that require abstract interpretation; and meaning interpretation, in areas that need elaboration and explanation in addition to translation. Coaching the interpreter in these different styles of interpretation can make the interpretive process more efficient and useful (Westermeyer 1990).

Clinical Assessment and Diagnosis

Psychiatric assessment results from a dynamic process that involves multiple levels of interaction between the patient (and sometimes the patient's family) and the clinician (Tseng 1997).

Experience of Distress by the Patient

A person experiences pain when he is hit; feels anxious if he is worried about something; becomes paranoid if he suspects that he is being persecuted by others; or feels sad if he has lost something significant to him. All these reactions to distress—which may be manifested as symptoms or signs—are subjective, experiential phenomena. However, it is clear that the source of the distress can be influenced by sociocultural factors. For instance, stress can be produced by culturally demanded performance. Stress can be created by culturally maintained beliefs. Stress can be generated by cultural restrictions of behavior, culture-supported attitudes, or other culture-related factors (Tseng 2001, pp. 128–136).

Perception of Problems by the Patient

After the experience of distress and the emergence of symptoms, the patient perceives and interprets the distressing experience. This psychological phenomenon is subject to the influence of cultural factors in addition to other variables, such as the patient's personality, knowledge, and psychological needs. Depending on how the problem is understood and perceived by the patient, he will show a secondary process of various reactions to the distress. In other words, the patient's perception of and reaction to the primary symptoms will add secondary symptoms that compound the clinical picture. The process of forming secondary symptoms is usually subject to cultural influences.

Presentation of Complaints or Illness by the Patient

The next step is the presentation of the complaints or illness by the patient to others—the process and art of "complaining." Analysis of this process has shown that the way the problem, symptom, or illness is presented or communicated to the clinician is based on the patient's (or his or her family's) orientation to illness, the meaning of the symptoms, motivation for help seeking, and culturally expected or sanctioned problem-presenting style. It is a combination of the results of these factors that affects the process of complaining. However, culture definitely plays a role in this complaining process.

For instance, patients of certain ethnic groups tend to make somatic complaints to their clinicians in their initial sessions at mental health clinics. This tendency requires careful understanding. There may be several alternative implications: a physical condition is the patient's primary concern; somatic symptoms are being used as socially recognized signals of illness; the symptoms constitute a culturally sanctioned prelude to revealing psychological problems; or the symptoms are a reflection of hypochondriacal traits that are shared by the group (Tseng 1975). Therefore, the nature of the somatic complaint needs to be carefully evaluated and understood rather than simply dealt with or labeled as a somatoform disorder.

Conversely, as mentioned earlier, a patient from another ethnic background might present many psychological problems to the therapist in the initial session, complaining that as a small child she was abused by some adult, was never adequately loved by her parents, and is now confused about her own identity, unclear about the meaning of life, and so on. It is necessary for the clinician to determine how much of this psychologized complaint may merely reflect the patient's learned behavior from public communication about patienthood and how much of it is really of primary concern. The performance of complaining or problem presentation is an art that does not directly reflect the distress or problem that the patient is experiencing. A dynamic interpretation and understanding are necessary.

Perception and Understanding of the Disorder by the Clinician

A clinician, as a cultural person and a professional, has his or her own ways of perceiving and understanding the complaints that are presented by the patient. The clinician's psychological sensitivity, cultural awareness, professional orientation, experience, and medical competence all act together to influence his or her assessment of the problems a patient has presented (Streltzer 1997). The cultural background of the clinician is a significant factor that deserves special attention, particularly when he or she is examining a patient with a different cultural background or one with which the clinician is unfamiliar. The clinician's style of interviewing, perception of and sensitivity toward pathology, and familiarity with the disorder under examination all influence his or her interaction with the patient, which in turn influences the outcome of the clinician's understanding of the disorder (Tseng et al. 1992).

Diagnosis and Categorization of the Disorder by the Clinician

The final step in the process of evaluation is making a clinical diagnosis. Determination of the appropriate clinical category for the diagnosis is influenced by the professional orientation of the clinician, the classification system used, and the purpose of making the diagnosis (Cooper et al. 1969; Jilek 1993; Tseng et al. 1992). In many societies, a clinician needs to take into consideration the social impact of diagnostic labeling on the patient and the family.

In sum, making a clinical assessment and diagnosis is a complex matter involving a dynamic process between the help seeker and the help provider. The assessment and diagnostic process is influenced in a variety of ways by the cultural background of the patient, as by that of the clinician. The clinician who is aware of how cultural factors affect each step in the process has a distinct advantage.

Conceptual Distinction Between Disease and Illness

To facilitate the understanding of transcultural medical practice, it has been proposed that a distinction be made between disease and illness (Eisenberg 1977). The term *disease* refers to a pathological condition or malfunction that is diagnosed by a doctor or folk healer. It is the clinician's conceptualization of the patient's problem, which derives from the paradigm of disease in which the clinician was trained. For example, a biomedically oriented psychiatrist is trained to diagnose brain disease; a psychoanalyst is trained to diagnose psychodynamic problems; and a folk healer might be trained to conceptualize and interpret such things as spirit possession or sorcery. For a medically oriented psychiatrist, the term *mental disease* is used to describe a pathological condition that can be grasped and comprehended from a medical point of view; it provides an objective and professional perspective on how the sickness may occur, how it is manifested, how it progresses, and how it ends.

In contrast, the term *illness* refers to the sickness that is experienced and perceived by the patient, including his or her subjective perception, experience, and interpretation of the suffering. Although the terms *disease* and *illness* are linguistically almost synonymous, they are purposely used differently to refer to two separate conditions. This usage is intended to illustrate that disease, as perceived by the healer or doctor, might not be similar to illness, as perceived and experienced by the person who is suffering. This artificial distinction is useful from a cultural perspective because it illustrates a potential gap between the healer (or doctor) and the help seeker (or patient) in viewing the problems. Although the biomedically oriented physician tends to assume that disease is a universal medical entity, from a medical-anthropological point of view all clinicians' diagnoses, as well as patients' illness experiences, are cognitive constructions based on cultural schemas. The potential gap between disease and illness is an area that deserves the clinician's attention and management in making his or her clinical assessment meaningful and useful, particularly in a cross-cultural situation.

Culture and Psychopathology

Culture substantially influences psychopathology (Tseng and Streltzer 1997). The various ways that culture contributes to psychopathology have been termed *pathogenetic, pathoplastic, pathoelaborating, pathofacilitating, pathodiscriminating,* and *pathoreactive effects* (Tseng 2001). Culture has less influence on organic mental disorders and major psychiatric disorders (functional psychoses) than on minor psychiatric disorders (neuroses) or substance abuse. Culture has a profound influence on culture-related specific syndromes or epidemic mental disorders (Tseng 2001).

Culture and Psychiatric Treatment

Psychiatric Treatment in General

In addition to socioeconomic and medical factors per se (including knowledge and theory), the mode of psychiatric treatment is also directly or indirectly influenced by cultural factors. For instance, the decision to follow a more biologically or a more psychologically oriented treatment model is subject to the patient's and the therapist's views on the usefulness of these models, and these views are based on their cultural attitudes and beliefs. Decisions regarding whether the patient should be treated in a closed institution with custodial care or in an open system in the community are greatly influenced by the family's and the community's attitudes toward mental illness.

Culture and Psychotherapy

Psychotherapy is greatly influenced by cultural factors (Tseng and Streltzer 2001). This is true of both the technical aspects and the theoretical and philosophical considerations of psychotherapy (Tseng 1995). This influence is discussed in detail in Chapter 11 (Culture and Psychotherapy).

Ethnicity, Race, and Drug Therapy

Genetic and other biological factors affect pharmacokinetic and pharmacodynamic processes. In addition, significant psychological factors—closely associated with social and cultural factors—influence the giving and receiving of medication. These issues are discussed in detail in Chapter 10 (Culture and Drug Therapy).

Conclusion

In this introductory chapter we have identified the variety of areas in which culture influences the clinical practice of psychiatry. The chapters that follow address how these cultural factors may be dealt with to provide culturally competent psychiatric care in different clinical settings (inpatient, outpatient, emergency, or liaison-consultation), for different problems (addiction or forensic), for different patient populations (child-adolescent or geriatric), and using different modes of psychiatric care (drug therapy or psychotherapy). The matter of cultural competence in clinical practice can be comprehensively addressed by examining psychiatric practice from the perspectives of different services for different patient populations with different clinical issues.

References

Bizi-Nathaniel S, Granec M, Colomb M: Psychotherapy of an Arab patient by a Jewish therapist in Israel during the Intifada. Am J Psychother 45:594–603, 1991

Brantley T: Racism and its impact on psychotherapy. Am J Psychiatry 140:1605–1608, 1983

Burke AW (ed): Transcultural psychiatry: racism and mental illness. Int J Soc Psychiatry 30 (1–2), 1984 (30th anniversary double edition)

Carter RT: The Influence of Race and Racial Identity in Psychotherapy: Toward a Racially Inclusive Model. New York, Wiley, 1995

Collins D, Dimsdale JE, Wilkins D: Consultation-liaison psychiatric utilization patterns in different cultural groups. Psychosom Med 54:240–245, 1992

Comas-Díaz L: Cross-cultural mental health treatment, in Clinical Guidelines in Cross-Cultural Mental Health. Edited by Comas-Díaz L, Griffith E. New York, Wiley, 1988, pp 335–361

Comas-Díaz L, Jacobsen FM: Ethnocultural transference and countertransference in the therapeutic dyad. Am J Orthopsychiatry 61:392–401, 1991

Cooper JE, Kendall RE, Gurland BJ, et al: Cross-national study of diagnosis of the mental disorders: some results from the first comparative investigation. Am J Psychiatry 125(suppl):21–29, 1969

Eisenberg L: Disease and illness: distinction between professional and popular ideas of sickness. Cult Med Psychiatry 1:9–23, 1977

Elderkin-Thompson V, Silver RC, Waitzkin H: When nurses double as interpreters: a study of Spanish-speaking patients in a U.S. primary care setting. Soc Sci Med 52:1343–1358, 2001

Foulks E: The concept of culture in psychiatric residency education. Am J Psychiatry 137:811–816, 1980

Griffith MS: The influences of race on the psychotherapeutic relationship. Psychiatry 40:27–40, 1977

Jilek WG: Traditional medicine relevant to psychiatry, in Treatment of Mental Disorders. Edited by Sartorius N, De Girolamo G, Andrews G, et al. Washington DC, American Psychiatric Press, 1993, pp 341–390

Kaplan S, Busner J: A note on racial bias in the admission of children and adolescents to state mental health facilities versus correctional facilities in New York. Am J Psychiatry 149:768–772, 1992

Kinzie D: Cultural aspects of psychiatric treatment with Indochinese refugees. Am J Soc Psychiatry 5:47–53, 1985

Lambley P, Cooper P: Psychotherapy and race: interracial therapy under apartheid. Am J Psychother 29:179–184, 1975

Leach MM, Harbin JJ: Psychological ethics codes: a comparison of twenty-four countries. Int J Psychol 32:181–192, 1997

Lee E (ed): Working With Asian Americans: A Guide for Clinicians. New York, Guilford, 1997

Littlewood R: Psychiatric diagnosis and racial bias: empirical and interpretative approaches. Soc Sci Med 34:141–149, 1992

Lu FG, Lim RF, Mezzich JE: Issues in the assessment and diagnosis of culturally diverse individuals, in American Psychiatric Press Review of Psychiatry, Vol 14. Edited by Oldham JM, Riba MB. Washington DC, American Psychiatric Press, 1995, pp 477–510

Marcos LR: Effects of interpreters on the evaluation of psychopathology in non-English-speaking patients. Am J Psychiatry 136:171–174, 1979

Moffic MS, Kendrick EA, Reid K: Cultural psychiatry education during psychiatric residency. J Psychiatr Educ 12:90–101, 1988

Neki JS, Joinet B, Hogan M, et al: The cultural perspective of therapeutic relationships: a viewpoint from Africa. Acta Psychiatr Scand 71:543–550, 1985

Nilchaikovit T, Hill JM, Holland JC: The effects of culture on illness behavior and medical care: Asian and American differences. Gen Hosp Psychiatry 15:41–50, 1993

Okasha A, Arboleda-Florez J, Sartorius N (ed): Ethics, Culture, and Psychiatry: International Perspectives. Washington DC, American Psychiatric Press, 2000

Paniagua FA: Assessing and Treating Culturally Diverse Clients: A Practical Guide, 2nd Edition. Thousand Oaks, CA, Sage, 1998

Pinderhughes E: Teaching empathy: ethnicity, race, and power at the cross-cultural treatment interface. Am J Soc Psychiatry 4:5–12, 1984

Sabshin M, Diesenhaus H, Wilkerson R: Dimensions of institutional racism in psychiatry. Am J Psychiatry 127:787–793, 1970

Siegel JM: A brief review of the effects of race in clinical service interactions. Am J Orthopsychiatry 44:555–562, 1974

Steere J, Dowdall T: On being ethical in unethical places: the dilemmas of South African clinical psychologists. Hastings Cent Rep 20:11–15, 1990

Stein HF: American Medicine as Culture. Boulder, CO, Westview Press, 1993

Streltzer J: Pain, in Culture and Psychopathology: A Guide to Clinical Assessment. Edited by Tseng WS, Streltzer J. New York, Brunner/Mazel, 1997, pp 87–100

Tseng WS: The nature of somatic complaints among psychiatric patients: the Chinese case. Compr Psychiatry 16:237–245, 1975

Tseng WS: Psychotherapy for the Chinese: cultural adjustment, in Psychotherapy for the Chinese, Vol II. Edited by Cheng LYC, Baxter H, Cheung FMC. Hong Kong, The Chinese University of Hong Kong, Department of Psychiatry, 1995, pp 1–22

Tseng WS: Overview: culture and psychopathology, in Culture and Psychopathology: A Guide to Clinical Assessment. Edited by Tseng WS, Streltzer J. New York, Brunner/Mazel, 1997, pp 1–27

Tseng WS: Handbook of Cultural Psychiatry. San Diego, CA, Academic Press, 2001

Tseng WS: The Clinician's Guide to Cultural Psychiatry. San Diego, CA, Academic Press, 2003

Tseng WS, Hsu J: Culture and psychotherapy, in Perspectives on Cross-Cultural Psychology. Edited by Marsella AJ, Tharp RG, Ciborowski TJ. New York, Academic Press, 1979, pp 333–345

Tseng WS, Streltzer J: Culture and Psychopathology: A Guide to Clinical Assessment. New York, Brunner/Mazel, 1997

Tseng WS, Streltzer J: Integration and conclusion, in Culture and Psychotherapy: A Guide for Clinical Practice. Edited by Tseng WS, Streltzer J. Washington, DC, American Psychiatric Press, 2001, pp 265–278

Tseng WS, Asai MH, Kitanishi KJ, et al: Diagnostic pattern of social phobia: comparison in Tokyo and Hawaii. J Nerv Ment Dis 180:380–385, 1992

Tseng WS, Ebata K, Kim KI, et al: Mental health in Asia: improvement and challenges. Int J Soc Psychiatry 47(1):8–23, 2001

Well K, Hough RL, Golding JM, et al: Which Mexican-Americans underutilize health services? Am J Psychiatry 144:918–922, 1987

Westermeyer J: The Psychiatric Care of Migrants: A Clinical Guide. Washington, DC, American Psychiatric Press, 1989

Westermeyer J: Working with an interpreter in psychiatric assessment and treatment. J Nerv Ment Dis 178:745–749, 1990

Yutrzenka BA: Making a case for training in ethnic and cultural diversity in increasing treatment efficacy. J Consult Clin Psychol 63:197–206, 1995

2

Culture and Inpatient Psychiatry

Francis G. Lu, M.D.

Inpatient psychiatry is a vital aspect of the psychiatric care continuum that has rapidly changed over the past 15 years. It has become more medically oriented with much shorter lengths of stay and is populated by increasingly poorer and more acutely ill patients (Druss et al. 1998; Jayaram et al. 1996; Summergrad 1994). In this context inpatient units have become the equivalent of the psychiatric intensive care unit (Beer et al. 2001). Staff members must rapidly establish rapport, gather clinical history, formulate the case, create a differential diagnosis, and construct a treatment plan with little margin for error. Given the nature of the 24-hour, multidisciplinary setting, such clinical processes take place in the context of a team or unit milieu, which requires an understanding of a systems approach. Issues to be considered include multidisciplinary staffing; milieu activities; family involvement; psychotherapy, pharmacotherapy, and disposition planning; and close interface with emergency services and outside agencies.

Studies in psychiatric inpatient care for ethnic minority populations indicate a disparity in utilization and diagnosis: African Americans and Native Americans are considerably more likely than Caucasian Americans to be hospitalized; Hispanic Americans and Asian Americans are less likely to be hospitalized (Snowden 1999). African Americans and Asian Americans are more likely to be diagnosed with the more severe disorder of schizophrenia and less likely to be diagnosed with a less severe mood disorder than are Caucasian Americans (American Psychiatric Association 2000). These disparities in utilization are also seen in other Western countries. In the United Kingdom, Commander and colleagues (1999) reported that Asian and black patients experienced more complex pathways and had higher levels of involvement with the police and compulsory detention than did Caucasians. Asian and black patients were less likely to perceive themselves as having a psychiatric problem or as needing to go into the hospital and expressed less satisfaction with the admission process. In Australia, Hassett and colleagues (1999) reported that elderly patients from non-English-speaking backgrounds were less likely to be admitted voluntarily and were less likely to be diagnosed with affective disorders.

Such disparities have led to increased attention to developing culturally competent inpatient services in the United States, beginning with the Asian Focus Unit in the Department of Psychiatry of the University of California, San Francisco, at San Francisco General Hospital in 1980 (Gee et al. 1999). Other specialized units for African Americans, Hispanic Americans, and Jewish Americans have also been described (Clark 1999; Herrera and Collazo 1999; Sublette and Trappler 2000). Guarnaccia (1999) outlined some of the cultural elements of such units from an anthropological perspective: 1) ethnic and cultural identity (complex and dynamic); 2) language; 3) material signs and symbols, events and celebrations, shared values; and 4) views of mental illness that may differ between the patient and the clinician. In this chapter, lessons learned from these special services have been distilled to provide the clinician with practical guidelines in the care of culturally diverse patients in inpatient units. This information is coupled with additional experiences from ordinary inpatient services that are characterized by caring for multiethnic patients in multicultural communities.

Inpatient Settings and Staff Relations

The successful provision of inpatient care does not occur in a vacuum; on the contrary, it is closely related to the way in which a unit's leadership works cooperatively with the clinical staff to model such collaborative relationships with outside agencies (Munich 2000). Typically, a chief psychiatrist and head nurse or nurse manager may co-lead a unit; their synergistic collaboration is essential for the success of the unit. Their cultural sensitivity is crucial to running a culturally relevant inpatient service. Depending on the number of beds, there might be additional psychiatrists.

In some states, psychologists are allowed medical staff privileges and can provide the nonmedical aspects of psychiatric attending care in addition to psychological testing. Nursing care by registered nurses and other nursing staff is typically divided into three shifts to cover 24 hours of service. The nursing staff have the most hands-on contact with patients, and their sensitivity, knowledge, and experience in working with patients of various ethnic and cultural backgrounds are key to culturally competent care. Social workers focus on assessment and therapy of family members and significant others in addition to post-hospital disposition planning. Occupational therapists provide many of the group vocational activities. In addition, other therapists, including art, drama, dance, and recreation therapists, may contribute to the multidisciplinary approach of inpatient care. Close support through formal and informal staff meetings and seamless communication are necessary for all of these disparate staff members to work together throughout the 24 hours. Typically, this is facilitated by a process of multidisciplinary team meetings several times a week to review the psychiatric history, discuss formulation and differential diagnosis, and decide on treatment and disposition plans.

A strategic plan for a culturally competent inpatient unit should inform such issues as needs assessment of the patients, staff recruitment and retention, policies, procedures, and training. Staffing should reflect the cultural needs of the patients that the unit serves. For example, if the admissions include patients with limited English proficiency, bilingual staff members, or at least trained interpreters who are able to speak the languages of the patient population, should be available. Regular inservice training should take place that includes a focus on cultural issues in clinical care. Staff members of multiethnic backgrounds will usually facilitate the cultural aspects of psychiatric care. The availability of cultural psychiatrists for consultation, and of resource persons with cultural knowledge of specific ethnic groups, will certainly contribute to a culturally competent treatment milieu.

Admission to a Psychiatric Unit

Implications of Psychiatric Hospitalization

Depending on how the patient, his family, and people in the community and in their original culture view mental disorders, the patient will have different attitudes and reactions to psychiatric hospitalization. If the patient comes from a society that holds a strong stigma against mental disorders, the patient will regard psychiatric hospitalization as a terrible thing, because he will now be regarded as a "crazy" person by his friends and by others. This would be particularly true if the hospital has an environment of poor quality and is filled with many very sick mental patients. Some patients might attempt to escape or even commit suicide if they perceive psychiatric hospitalization as the end of their lives (Jones 2003).

In contrast to this, if the community does not have a strong bias against mental disorders and if the quality of the psychiatric ward is better than the patient's own living conditions at home, the patient might be pleased to be hospitalized and enjoy the better food and facilities. Some patients (particularly those who are homeless), having learned to complain that they are suicidal, may even show up at emergency rooms to get immediate attention and be hospitalized. Such patients know that they can enjoy a comfortable bed and warm food for a few days. Thus, providing relevant clinical care requires attention to the different reactions by patients of diverse cultural backgrounds to psychiatric hospitalization (Tseng 2003).

Different Qualities of Service

Directly influenced by socioeconomic factors—including payment and the patient's financial condition, as well as the attitudes and degree of stigma associated with severe mental illness—the quality of inpatient care varies greatly among different societies and may be different even within the same society. Some facilities are very comfortable, even at the luxury level, whereas some are terribly deficient with regard to comfort. Setting up conditions in the hospital such that there is suitability for medical treatment while maintaining the living standards of the community and ensuring that there is not too big a gap between them (i.e., hospital conditions are not too luxurious or too poor) is very important. If the conditions are too poor, patients will be reluctant to be hospitalized, but if they are too luxurious, patients will be reluctant to be discharged back into the community.

Cultural Accommodations

It is not only the quality of service that requires attention and adjustment toward the community to meet the needs of psychiatric patients; a psychiatric ward also needs to be set up in such a way that it will fit the patients' diverse cultural backgrounds. For example, one important consideration is to provide, if at all possible, various kinds of ethnic foods to meet patients' tastes.

Providing a facility and religious personnel to offer various kinds of religious counseling and ceremonies to suit multifaith patient populations also deserves attention. The major thrust is a cultural concern for the environment and the institutional system in which patient care is to be provided.

Language Barriers as Problems

Problems in Communication

Communication through language is an important aspect of medical practice in general, and this is particularly critical in psychiatric practice. Soliciting the necessary clinical history and clarifying symptoms depend on communication in psychiatric practice. It is a serious problem when the patient does not speak a language that is understood by the physician or health care workers.

Many patients who are psychotic or severely depressed already have problems expressing their ideas and feelings, and they may be less talkative or show symptoms of autistic thinking. This problem is compounded when there is a language barrier.

Limitations of Translation

If there is a language barrier, translation is needed. Obtaining professionally correct translation and culturally relevant interpretation is a matter of skill that deserves special attention. It is desirable to have interpreters for various languages. There is also a need for psychiatric training for professional interpreters to permit more meaningful and accurate translation to take place (see Chapter 1, Introduction: Culture and Psychiatry). However, no matter how well trained and skillful the interpreter, there are always limitations to translation. It is a critical challenge to understand a patient's mind and behavior beyond the semantic level to reach the meanings behind his words.

Case 1: A Chinese Patient With the Ability to Foresee Things

Mr. Tang, a young Chinese patient, was on his way from the United States back to China when he became excited and acted strangely on the plane. He shouted to the flight attendant that the pilot needed to stop the flight, because he could foresee that a terrible accident would happen if the airplane continued to fly. Under the impression that the passenger was experiencing a mental breakdown, the pilot made an emergency landing, and Mr. Tang was sent to a hospital for psychiatric care. After his admission, his family in China was notified, and within a couple of days his elder brother arrived, intending to escort Mr. Tang immediately back to his home country. Because Mr. Tang spoke only limited English and his elder brother hardly spoke English at all, a Chinese-speaking translator was called when the psychiatrist had a joint meeting with the elder brother and the patient. The psychiatrist tried to explain to the elder brother that Mr. Tang was still mentally very sick and was not in any condition to take a flight. The interpreter faithfully translated into Chinese to the elder brother that the patient was still very "crazy" and the airline would not allow a "psychotic" patient on the airplane. The elder brother explained that his patient-brother had a special ability to foresee things and insisted that there was nothing wrong with him mentally. He tried to explain through the interpreter that, actually, he himself also had this special ability. From his forehead, he could radiate out a magic beam and read other people's minds—including the psychiatrist's. After hearing the interpreter's word-for-word translation, the psychiatrist was at a loss, not knowing how to make sense of what the elder brother had said. Finally, a Chinese-speaking cultural psychiatrist was consulted. After an interview was conducted in Chinese, it was concluded that the elder brother had a mental disorder as well. It was a rare case of *folie a deux*. Mr. Tang and his elder brother shared the delusion of telepathy, believing that they had a special mental ability to foresee things.

Clinical Assessment and Diagnosis

Psychological Testing

Psychiatrists and clinical psychologists sometimes use various kinds of psychological instruments to measure patients' psychological condition and assess psychopathology. Even when the questionnaire is translated into different languages, the cross-cultural validity of psychological instruments is subject to question. Determining the extent to which translated tests are applicable and culturally equivalent is still a challenge subject to investigation (Brislin 2000).

For instance, in a survey of Puerto Ricans, it was found that the Diagnostic Interview Schedule, the commonly used instrument designed for the Epidemiologic Catchment Area study, had to be modified in the interpretations of items concerning psychotic experiences (Guarnaccia et al. 1992). Because of the cultural proclivity toward belief in spirits, visions, voices, and presentiments, many features of Puerto Rican culture had to be incorporated into mental health assessments to correct for exaggerated attributions of psychotic symptoms. In a survey for bipolar disorders among the Amish people, it was reported that the operationalization of manic symptoms—such as buying dresses, sexual promiscuity, and reckless driving—was not applicable to the Old Order Amish (Egeland et al. 1983). These reports illustrated that careful interpretation is needed in the cross-cultural application of psychological measurements and that cultural adjustments are often necessary.

Mental Status Examination

Through clinical interviews a psychiatrist tries to clarify the chief complaint and to obtain a history of the present illness, family history, and psychiatric history. Beyond this, the psychiatrist usually carries out a mental status examination in either a formal or an informal way. For such an examination, psychiatrists are taught how to ask questions in certain ways and to examine various aspects of mental function, such as orientation, memory, cognition, affect, and perception. In the examination of patients of diverse cultural backgrounds, the formal or stylized mental status examination needs proper cultural adjustments. This is particularly true of examinations of psychotic patients.

For instance, when asking a patient to explain certain proverbs to examine the patient's comprehension of and ability for abstract thinking and style of thinking process, the psychiatrist needs to know to what extent the patient is familiar with the proverbs presented to him. Commonly used proverbs such as "A rolling stone gathers no moss" and "The grass is always greener on the other side of the fence" are Anglo-Saxon in origin and may not be familiar to non-Western patients. Conversely, Eastern proverbs such as "Ten years' cultivation for a monk, *amitofu* in one morning" (implying that a single mistake can ruin all of life's efforts) and "To lose some is to make a big gain" are likely to be unfamiliar to most Western patients. Selecting appropriate proverbs to use in an examination requires cultural consideration; otherwise, incorrect interpretations and conclusions will result.

When inquiring about the presence or absence of auditory hallucinations, to ask, "Do you hear any 'voices'?" may be sufficient for patients who know what it means to hear "voices" (auditory hallucinations) but could be easily misunderstood as an inquiry about hearing ability to a patient who is not familiar with the way psychiatrists ask for information.

Some Problematic Psychotic Symptoms

From a cultural perspective, clinical assessments are difficult to perform and diagnoses are difficult to make when they relate to certain kinds of psychotic symptoms, such as bizarre or inappropriate behavior, delusions, and disorientation.

It is generally difficult to make an assessment as to whether or not a thought is "bizarre," behavior is "strange," or affect is "inappropriate," because such judgments need to be based on "reality." However, reality is difficult to grasp if the examiner is unfamiliar with the "reality" in which the patient is living. Collateral information from family members or friends can be used for making such judgments.

Judgments on "delusions" are based on the presence of "false" beliefs not endorsed or shared by other people. However, what is true and false needs careful assessment based on social reality. This is particularly true if the delusion is related to religious or sexual matters. Distinguishing between "normally accepted and group-shared religious beliefs" and "individually based pathological religious beliefs" can be very tricky. If there is a problem in communication, without proper background information and clarification such a symptom is difficult to evaluate and judge.

In a similar way, in evaluating erotic delusions and those relating to sexual harassment, it may also be difficult to distinguish between what actually happened and the patient's delusional interpretation. It will always be helpful to look into whether or not there are other kinds of psychotic symptoms present. It will be useful to check with the family and friends of the patient and with people in the community when attempting to understand and interpret the content of the patient's delusions. If it is clear that the content of the delusions is relatively bizarre, the clinician will be better able to make an assessment.

Culture-Related Specific Clinical Pictures

It is often difficult for clinicians to make clinical diagnoses if they are unfamiliar or inexperienced with certain groups of disorders. For instance, Caucasian American psychiatrists are less experienced nowadays with dissociated or possessed disorders because patients with such disorders are becoming very unusual in Western societies, whereas Asian psychiatrists are less familiar with multiple personality disorders or various kinds of substance abuse or sexual disorders because patients with those disorders rarely appear in psychiatric care facilities in Asia.

If the clinical condition belongs to a so-called culture-specific syndrome, such as koro (an anxiety attack resulting from the folk belief that excessive shrinking of the penis into the abdomen will cause death), latah (a transient dissociative attack provoked by startling), or amok (indiscriminate, mass homicidal attacks in reaction to stress or loss), many clinicians may have difficulty making a relevant assessment and judgment (Tseng 2001).

Many folk terms—such as *voodoo death, ataque de nervios* (an attack of nerves), *susto* (loss of soul), or *hwabyung* (fire sickness)—are used by laypersons from different ethnic groups to describe certain distressing experiences. Determining whether these terms describe a culture-specific syndrome or indicate signs and symptoms of a mental disorder is a basic differential diagnostic assessment that clinicans must consider. In other words, clinical experiences and familiarity with disorders will certainly influence clinical competence in making a proper diagnosis. This is also true for psychotic patients in inpatient settings.

Case 2: A Korean Woman With "Fire Sickness"

Mrs. Kim, a young Korean woman, was brought by her parents for psychiatric care. They reported that recently she tended to cry and failed to take care of herself. Her parents suspected that Mrs. Kim was being mistreated by her husband and mother-in-law and that she had *hwabyung* (fire sickness). According to her parents' folk belief, a woman with emotional problems who was full of resentment and hate and was unable to deal with her psychological pain would experience fire sickness. Mrs. Kim's parents were particularly unhappy that their son-in-law did not take good care of their daughter and was even not enthusiastic about providing her with medical care.

When Mrs. Kim's husband was interviewed, he denied any mistreatment by him or his parents. He revealed that when Mrs. Kim was young, before she married him, she had had a psychiatric breakdown and had been treated by a psychiatrist. He said that after their marriage several years ago, his wife was found to have mood swings and occasionally became very depressed. It was concluded that Mrs. Kim had a mood disorder, rather than fire sickness associated with emotional hardship or stress as conceptualized in the folk interpretation.

Patient's Behavior in the Unit

Understanding Cultural Behavior

To provide proper assessment and management, the professional needs to observe and understand a patient's behavior. This is especially true in inpatient settings, where the staff will have an opportunity to observe and interact with the patient. Determining whether the patient's behavior is strange or bizarre or is culturally syntonic can be a challenge for mental health workers. The following case is an example of this challenge.

Case 3: A Muslim Patient Who Refused to Eat Pork

Mr. Sumarato, an Indonesian sailor, had a mental breakdown and was brought from his ship to a nearby Chinese harbor for emergency care. Subsequently, Mr. Sumarato was hospitalized in a Chinese psychiatric ward, with the diagnosis of acute delusional disorder. The paranoid condition manifested while he was on the ship. According to his captain, Mr. Sumarato believed that his fellow sailors and the captain were plotting to persecute him.

On the ward, Mr. Sumarato refused to eat certain foods. The Chinese psychiatric staff interpreted his behavior as reflecting his suspicion that the food was poisoned. He also exhibited what the staff interpreted as "bizarre" behavior, kneeling down on the ground and bowing in a certain direction three or four times a day. After consulting with a cultural expert, it was disclosed that the Indonesian patient, based on his Muslim religious beliefs, was careful not to eat pork (it was considered an unclean meat) and that he was performing his daily routine of worshipping God (Allah) when he was kneeling down and bowing toward the holy site of Mecca. He was certainly preoccupied by his persecutory delusions, continuing to talk about how dangerous it was for him on the ship, where his fellow sailors were trying to kill him. However, not eating certain food and performing certain behaviors of worship had nothing to do with his persecutory delusions. He was merely faithfully observing his religious beliefs. The Chinese staff were unfamiliar with the Muslim religion and had difficulty distinguishing between cultural behavior and psychotic behavior.

Ethnic Identity Issues

Ethnic identity issues may be observed in ordinary people in their daily lives. They may surface as prominent issues for some patients when they become mentally ill, and ethnic identity confusion may become part of their clinical picture. For example, a Laotian schizophrenic patient, feeling hurt after being rejected by his family in Laos, overidentified with America. In his psychotic condition, he denied being of Laotian heritage and refused to use his Laotian name, using his American name instead. On the ward, he always wore a an American flag pin and a red, white, and blue necktie (a symbol of America) to emphasize that he was an American. Despite his distinctly Asian face, he always pointed to Caucasian American people in magazines, claiming they were his parents (Locke 2003). Conversely, an American patient, after being abused and rejected by his American parents, experienced welcoming treatment in Asia while he was in the service. When he become psychotic, he developed the delusional belief that he was a descendant of Genghis Khan and denied his American ancestry.

In relations between patients and staff members, certain transferences may occur, which need proper attention and management. Sometimes the transference is related to ethnic issues; this is regarded as "ethnic transference." Psychotic ethnic transference may be observed in some patients in inpatient settings. The following is a typical example.

Case 4: An American Patient Who Accused Her Psychiatrist of Being "Vietcong"

Mrs. Waldon, a Caucasian American patient, was admitted to a psychiatric hospital for an acute mental illness, with delusional tendencies and other psychotic features. She was assigned for care to an Asian American psychiatrist. In her psychotic condition, the patient shouted at the psychiatrist: "You are Vietcong! Communist! Go back to Vietnam! Don't touch me, otherwise I will kill you!" In Mrs. Waldon's paranoid state she became very aggressive, picking up objects to throw at the psychiatrist. Several sessions of electroconvulsive therapy were administered to treat her delusional condition, and her agitation subsided remarkably. After she improved, Mrs. Waldon related very well with the psychiatrist and even remarked that he was one of the best doctors she had ever encountered. Apparently, Mrs. Waldon did not remember having misidentified him as Vietcong.

Treatment Issues

Drug Treatment

Besides electroconvulsive therapy, biological treatment in the form of medication is a primary therapeutic approach for psychotic inpatients. Ethnic factors can influence psychopharmacological response, which in turn shapes the optimal therapeutic dosage and severity of side effects (Ruiz 2000). Due to pharmacokinetic differences, therapeutic dosages are more likely to need considerable adjustment for some ethnic groups, such as Asian and Native American people, in contrast to Caucasian groups, which were more likely to be involved in the original research that determined dosage recommendations (see Chapter 10, Culture and Drug Therapy). In addition, side effects and their severity need proper attention and assessment; otherwise, they will significantly affect compliance with treatment.

In addition to pharmacological issues, the psychology of prescribing and receiving medication often influences drug response, and cultural issues can form a large part of this psychology. Patients will respond differently, with different adherence results, even to the same medication prescribed by different therapists who have different ways of giving medication.

Therapeutic Activities

In addition to drug treatment, various therapeutic programs are often provided in the psychiatric ward. These might include occupational therapy, recreational therapy, group therapy, and so on. On the basis of their knowledge and previous behavior patterns, patients of various ethnic or cultural backgrounds may respond differently to these different therapeutic activities.

Patients from societies where people are not used to expressing their feelings or examining their minds in front of others might not appreciate ward meetings or group therapy with their peer patients. Their behavior may be misinterpreted as being "asocial" or "passive" and "withdrawn." Actually, these patients may respond better to activity-oriented occupational therapy than to talking therapy in a group setting. This applies to music or dance therapy. Besides individual differences, there are also ethnic differences in preference for special activities.

In many inpatient settings, occupational therapy is useful for assessing a patient's behavior and level of function, promoting an active life and socialization, or preparing the patient for occupational rehabilitation. From a cultural point of view, it would be helpful if the patient had a wide selection of occupational activities that were familiar. This would make the patient feel more comfortable and more interested in engaging in them. This also applies to other therapeutic activities, again including music and dance therapy.

Working With the Family

Theoretically, it is important to involve the family in the process of care of the patient during hospitalization. It offers the therapist and staff an opportunity to observe how the patient relates to family members and how the family members treat the patient. Most important, involvement of the family provides an opportunity to educate the family in how to care for the psychotic patient. This improves the patient's prognosis after discharge from the hospital and return to the family.

Nevertheless, how much the family participates in the care of a psychiatric patient in a ward setting varies from society to society. In developing societies, in which family relations are emphasized, the family is commonly allowed to live with the patient day and night, working with the staff to care for their relative. In contrast, in societies (typically developed ones) in which family relations are not as highly valued due to a medical culture that believes visitors will interfere with the treatment program, friends or family members are allowed to visit a patient only at certain times under strict rules. Consequently, the degree and nature of family involvement in the care of the patient varies greatly. From a cultural perspective, there is a need to balance what is expected by the culture of the patient and family with the medical culture that is imposed on them. Inviting the family to join in the treatment planning and discussing ways of caring for the patient will be useful in many circumstances. This is indicated by the following case.

Case 5: A Hispanic Girl Who Lost Her Soul

Maria, an adolescent girl, was brought by her Hispanic parents to a mental health clinic for care. Several months before, she had been found wandering around talking to herself and laughing inappropriately. Her parents thought that their daughter must be experiencing *susto* (loss of soul) and tried to consult local healers to regain her soul. After attending several ceremonial sessions with a local healer, Maria did not show any improvement. Finally, as a last resort, Maria was brought to see a psychiatrist in the community mental health clinic. With a diagnosis of schizophrenia, she was hospitalized for treatment. During her hospitalization, her family visited almost every day. The staff took the opportunity to invite the family to participate in family sessions with the treating psychiatrist. The psychiatrist explained to the family that Maria had "lost her soul," causing her to act strangely, and it would take a while to regain it. It was explained that the medication (an antipsychotic) that was prescribed for Maria would help her soul stay in her and not wander about. It was suggested to the parents that it was very important that Maria keep taking the medicine, even after her discharge. This culture-adjusted explanation of the girl's sickness and the instructions given to the family were well received.

Suggestions for Clinical Practice

1. *Provide a culturally sensitive and competent unit setting.* Associated with advances in cultural psychiatry, it has become clear that cultural competence is necessary in psychiatric practice, even in the care of severely ill mental patients in inpatient settings. In addition to medical issues, it is also necessary to pay attention to cultural aspects to fit the care to the diverse cultural backgrounds of the patients. This is not only true in the design of the facilities where treatment takes place but also in the process of clinical assessment, diagnosis, treatment, and care.

2. *Provide a multiethnic staff for patients of various cultures.* To serve patients of diverse ethnic and cultural backgrounds, it is desirable to have staff members with multiethnic backgrounds who understand the essence and importance of cultural dimensions in our lives and in the lives of mentally ill persons. The availability of well-trained interpreters of various languages will be helpful to provide culturally geared mental health care. An effort should at least be made to locate cultural experts when they might be helpful in the treatment of patients of particular ethnic or cultural backgrounds.

Regular in-service training should take place, not only to update medical knowledge and skill, but also to focus on cultural issues in clinical care. Sharing and learning about various cultural systems will enhance cultural sensitivity, knowledge, and empathy—the core of cultural competence.

3. *Make culture-appropriate clinical assessments and diagnoses.* The Outline for Cultural Formulation in Appendix I of DSM-IV-TR (American Psychiatric Association 2000) provides a concise method for making such assessments. All clinicians should have a basic awareness that the process and results of clinical assessment and diagnosis are subject to various factors, including culture. Culture-relevant adjustments should be made when assessing patients' psychopathologies and psychological problems. This is true for psychological testing, clinical interviews, and formal mental status examinations.

4. *Make ethnically appropriate adjustments to drug therapy.* When administering drug therapy one needs to take into consideration the ethnic background of the patient. In determining the proper dosage for treatment, the patient's ethnic background—as well as his or her age and body weight and the nature and severity of psychopathology—needs to be considered to achieve effective results with as few side effects as possible.

In addition, understanding the psychology of giving and receiving medication—not only from the individual's perspective, but also from the perspective of the patient's culture—increases the likelihood of a successful response.

5. *Ensure active involvement of the family in the care of the patient.* The family of the patient should be involved as much as possible in the course of treatment. The nature of the patient's mental disorder, the strategies of treatment, and the principles of care should be explained to the family, and at the same time their input and participation in the care of the patient should be invited. The family is the basic unit of social life and support for the patient. Treating an individual patient is not enough; the whole family should be involved. This may be critical for people with cultures that emphasize the importance of the family.

References

American Psychiatric Association: Diagnostic and Statistical Manual of Mental Disorders, 4th Edition, Text Revision. Washington, DC, American Psychiatric Association, 2000

Beer MD, Pereira SM, Paton C (eds): Psychiatric Intensive Care. London, Greenwich Medical Media, 2001

Brislin RW: Some methodological concerns in intercultural and cross-cultural research, in Understanding Culture's Influence on Behavior, 2nd Edition. Edited by Brislin RW. Fort Worth, TX, Harcourt, 2000, pp 425–448

Clark M: Development of a client-centered inpatient service for African-Americans, in Cross Cultural Psychiatry. Edited by Herrera JM, Lawson WB, Sramek JJ. New York, Wiley, 1999, pp 287–293

Commander MJ, Cochrane R, Sashidharan SP, et al: Mental health care for Asian, black and white patients with non-affective psychoses: pathways to the psychiatric hospital, in-patient and after-care. Soc Psychiatry Psychiatr Epidemiol 34:484–491, 1999

Druss BG, Bruce ML, Jacobs SC, et al: Trends over a decade for a general hospital psychiatric unit. Adm Policy Ment Health 25:427–435, 1998

Egeland JA, Gaviria M, Pathak D, et al: Amish study, III: the impact of cultural factors on diagnosis of bipolar illness. Am J Psychiatry 140:67–71, 1983

Gee K, Du N, Akiyama K, et al: The Asian Focus Unit at UCSF: an 18-year perspective, in Cross Cultural Psychiatry. Edited by Herrera JM, Lawson WB, Sramek JJ. New York, Wiley, 1999, pp 275–285

Guarnaccia P: Anthropological issues on ethnic units, in Cross Cultural Psychiatry. Edited by Herrera JM, Lawson WB, Sramek JJ. New York, Wiley, 1999, pp 303–312

Guarnaccia PJ, Guevara-Ramos LM, Gonzales G, et al: Cross-cultural aspects of psychotic symptoms in Puerto Rico. Res Community Ment Health 7:99–110, 1992

Hassett A, George K, Harrigan S: Admissions of elderly patients from English-speaking and non-English-speaking backgrounds to an inpatient psychogeriatric unit. Aust N Z J Psychiatry 33:576–582, 1999

Herrera J, Collazo Y: The effectiveness of a culturally sensitive milieu on hospitalized Hispanic patients, in Cross Cultural Psychiatry. Edited by Herrera JM, Lawson WB, Sramek JJ. New York, Wiley, 1999, pp 295–302

Jayaram G, Tien AY, Sullivan P, et al: Elements of a successful short-stay inpatient psychiatric service. Psychiatr Serv 47:407–412, 1996

Jones L: Case 1: an elderly Asian man patient committed suicide after admission to a psychiatric hospital, in Clinician's Guide to Cultural Psychiatry. Edited by Tseng WS. San Diego, CA, Academic Press, 2003, p 262

Locke S: Case 1: a Laotian man who overidentified with America, in Clinician's Guide to Cultural Psychiatry. Edited by Tseng WS. San Diego, CA, Academic Press, 2003, p 35

Munich RL: Leadership and restructured roles: the evolving inpatient treatment team. Bull Menninger Clin 64:482–493, 2000

Ruiz P (ed): Ethnicity and Psychopharmacology. Washington, DC, American Psychiatric Press, 2000

Snowden L: Psychiatric inpatient care and ethnic minority populations, in Cross Cultural Psychiatry. Edited by Herrera JM, Lawson WB, Sramek JJ. New York, Wiley, 1999, pp 261–273

Sublette E, Trappler B: Cultural sensitivity training in mental health: treatment of Orthodox Jewish psychiatric inpatients. Int J Soc Psychiatry 46:122–134, 2000

Summergrad P: Medical psychiatric units and the roles of the inpatient psychiatric service in the general hospital. Gen Hosp Psychiatry 16:20–31, 1994

Tseng WS: Handbook of Cultural Psychiatry. San Diego, CA, Academic Press, 2001

Tseng WS: Clinician's Guide to Cultural Psychiatry. San Diego, CA, Academic Press, 2003

3

Culture and Outpatient Psychiatry

J. David Kinzie, M.D.
Paul K. Leung, M.D.

In this chapter we discuss the processes involved in the care of psychiatric outpatients when cultural factors are important to treatment. We have worked for more than two decades in special clinics dedicated to treating patients from Asia, Southeast Asia, Eastern Europe, North Africa, and Central America who mostly came to the hosting society of the United States as war refugees (Kinzie 1986; Kinzie et al. 1980). Besides the transcultural effects of migration between countries and cultures, these patients and their families have to struggle with the problems of language in adapting to the new society, the massive psychological trauma that they have encountered in the past, and continuous suffering from the sequelae of the stress that they have experienced. Working with these groups of refugees has been an unusual clinical experience characterized by extreme circumstances and patients with language problems associated with transcultural migration and posttraumatic stress problems. It offers the opportunity to examine how cultural issues affect the care of psychiatric outpatients in extreme situations. We hope that the knowledge and insight obtained from these unique clinical experiences can be generalized and extended into general practice for evaluating and treating ethnically and culturally different patients in outpatient services.

Basic Awareness: Working in Three Different "Cultures"

The Culture of the Psychiatrist

As pointed out in Chapter 1 (Introduction: Culture and Psychiatry), the psychiatrist belongs to a medical culture based on medical training, hospital and professional affiliations, a shared code of ethics, and multiple regulatory agencies controlling and monitoring his or her professional behavior. The values of this medical culture include individualism, mastery of nature and disease, and a future orientation (Kinzie 1985). A shared belief is that aggressive treatment can modulate most conditions. For psychiatrists, common obstacles to practice include third-party payers who limit payments, require increased documentation, and limit the number of treatment sessions. Practice is also subject to oversight by medical boards and licensing authorities. In addition to keeping abreast of the multiple advances in biological psychiatry, the psychiatrist is encouraged to be responsible for some of the medical problems (Pomeroy et al. 2002), spiritual needs (Boehnlein 2000), and—especially now—cultural assessment of their patients (Group for the Advancement of Psychiatry 2002). It is not surprising that psychiatrists feel besieged and overwhelmed. Treating the culturally different (sometimes for reduced fees), along with other pressures, may strain the psychiatrist's understanding and empathic capacities.

The Culture of the Psychiatric Patient

Most psychiatric patients face their first meeting with a psychiatrist apprehensively. The decision to seek psychiatric help, voluntarily or under pressure, was made after much deliberation and thought involving the fear of "going crazy" or "losing one's mind," which is often associated with hospitalization. The patient may also fear that the psychiatrist will force (or, more accurately, advocate) the use of medicine and will discount the patient's subjective complaints of not being understood. At the other extreme are fears of being understood too well—problems, fantasies, illegal or immoral behavior, drug abuse, and instances of domestic violence may be discovered. Ambivalence, wanting both to open up and to keep one's secret, is a core issue for patients. A special issue of concern is the possibility that the doctor will overlook physical problems—such as a brain tumor or abnormal chemistry—that affect behavior. The real and imaginary fears add to the psychiatric problem that led the patient to seek help in the first place. For most patients without adequate insurance coverage, the financial cost is also an issue.

The Culture of Culturally Different Groups

As difficult as it is for patients to seek psychiatric care, it is more difficult for those who are members of a minority group, are disadvantaged, or are from outside the mainstream culture. They often have no idea what to expect—except fear and uncertainty—and in fact they have historically been discriminated against in the mental health system (Moffic and Kinzie 1996). Moreover, they have an image of a passive, silent therapist, rather than a normal doctor who will take a history and perform a physical examination. The fear of being labeled crazy is ubiquitous. For many close-knit extended families, such as in most Asian cultures, a crazy person reflects in a shameful manner on the entire family. Clearly, making and keeping the appointment with a psychiatrist is done only after much pain and probably disruption.

Many cultural and experiential factors influence the patient's presentation. A major one is a fear of being put down because of dress or appearance. A clear example is a conservatively dressed Muslim woman who felt exceptionally conspicuous after the events of September 11, 2001. The patient's deep sense of being scrutinized and discriminated against was present even in psychiatric consultation rooms. There is also the fear of not being understood, such as among Muslim men with multiple wives, Gypsy women with lack of education, or Buddhists who need to perform a ceremony for their deceased parents. There is also a fear of deep family secrets being revealed, such as domestic violence in a Catholic family, alcoholism in a Muslim family, or having given up a daughter for prostitution in a poor Asian family.

Disadvantaged patients also have practical problems that are often neglected by the middle-class psychiatrist. Such effects on therapy might include not having enough money even for a modest copayment for medicine; the inability to read English and being unable to follow the instructions on the medicine bottle; not having enough money for bus fare to get to the appointment; and the difficulty for a non-English-speaking single mother to obtain a babysitter, causing missed appointments.

Another preconception of culturally different patients comes from their contacts with general physicians. It is increasingly clear that primary care physicians need to see many patients and to concentrate on specific complaints, and they have little time or sustained interest in their patients' total health. This is especially apparent for people who speak little or no English, cannot articulate their concerns, and are not encouraged to ask questions. They feel put down, ignored, and poorly treated and often have not received any relief of their symptoms. Many patients begin to expect a hurried, superficial visit with its accompanying disappointments.

A special issue that clinicians need to know about is the high likelihood of massive trauma in some ethnic groups (Boehnlein and Kinzie 1995; Kinzie et al. 1990). The effects of war, ethnic cleansing, and guerrilla activities are well known and should be addressed in refugees from Indochina, Bosnia, Somalia, and Central America. The effects of domestic violence, drug-related violence at home and in schools, and sexual assaults should also be approached. These are very sensitive issues that have their own associated numbness, avoidance, and amnesia, which make it difficult for patients to remember and to discuss.

Use of Counselors as Interpreters

Many patients from other cultures speak limited or no English. The treatment of these people often requires the use of interpreters. Providing mental health services through an interpreter is a complicated and difficult task. In our specialty clinics we accomplish this by training our own mental health counselors from each culture we serve. They not only act as interpreters but are also trained in case management.

Our training program is described here to emphasize the problems and values of interpreters. Our policy has always been to recruit counselors from a particular ethnicity and culture for their personal qualities—warmth, genuineness, and respect within their own culture—so that others in that culture can feel comfortable discussing personal information. Their knowledge of psychiatric disorders and their treatment is not important at first. In initial sessions, the new counselors act solely as interpreters. They are instructed to interpret word for word with the corresponding affect for both the patient and the psychiatrist. This is both necessary to evaluate the patient's thought organization and very difficult to do. The interpreters find it hard to be just a conduit for information and often feel the need to explain the patient or the doctor or to distance themselves from either. Another recurring issue is that a patient may bring up very disturbing material that resonates with the interpreter's own life. Reliving personal traumas occasionally makes it difficult to perform the role effectively—or sometimes even at all.

Case 1: A Counselor Reacts to a Patient's Traumatic Story

Mr. Seng, a young Cambodian, joined the program as a counselor trainee. On one occasion he was observing the psychiatrist and his supervisor evaluating a Cambodian woman. The evaluation was proceeding normally, and this type of interview had been performed many times by the treatment team. The woman was telling her story about the torture she had experienced at the hands of the Khmer Rouge camp guards and how she had witnessed the executions of campmates who had stolen food from others. As she was recounting the number of family members who died under the regime, Mr. Seng picked up a magazine, flipped through it, and actively avoided the patient and her suffering. This greatly annoyed the physician and the supervisor, and Mr. Seng was asked to put the magazine down. Mr. Seng was understandably embarrassed but could not offer an explanation for the unprofessional behavior.

Many years afterward, when Mr. Seng had long been successfully integrated into the program, he reluctantly disclosed his own traumatic past. He had lost seven of his immediate family members in the Khmer Rouge camps, and he was a survivor of a concentration camp.

Many immigrant mental health professionals came from the same war-ravaged lands as their clients. They have likely suffered the same types of traumatic experiences as the patients who are seeking help from them. Sometimes the only psychological defense these professionals have is to distance themselves either physically or emotionally from their patients, often doing it without self-awareness.

A Training Program for Counselors

The training of counselors in our program is a long process. It begins by observing other counselors' and psychiatrists' interactions. There is also supervision by senior counselors. A seminar program, taught by both senior counselors and psychiatrists, is given annually. It involves charting, regulations, DSM-IV-TR diagnoses (American Psychiatric Association 2000), and counseling technique. After receiving training, the new counselor performs mental health assessments, including history and provisional diagnosis, under supervision. This provides a background for the psychiatrist's formal assessment, which is the primary document for diagnosis and treatment. Most counselors also lead a group, emphasizing skills training and socialization. This is an important treatment issue in overcoming isolation, but it is not group therapy per se. The counselors also aid in helping the patients with medical appointments and obtaining financial and immigration assistance. At all times they are interpreters for the psychotherapist, and they are not to interfere with the special therapeutic relationship between patient and doctor. The counselor sometimes provides information learned from contact with the patient or provides cultural information that clarifies treatment. Overall, it takes about 4 years of training for a new counselor to be effective in the multiple roles. Ongoing supervision, individually and in groups, and a supportive work environment help with counter-transference feelings and the possibility of burnout (Boehnlein et al. 1998).

Working With Interpreters

For psychiatrists with trained interpreter/counselors, the issues are different. First, it is important to assess the interpreter's competence and comfort with mental health issues. Some are so inadequately trained or insensitive that questions must be simple and the psychiatrist must give nonverbal indications of support. If the interpreter can follow the instructions, it is useful to ask him or her to interpret exactly what is said—not to summarize or, more often, try to make sense of it. The psychiatrist should keep the focus on the patient and avoid making side comments to the interpreter because he or she speaks English.

With the interpretation process there is a great deal of time when neither the patient nor the psychiatrist is speaking. This is valuable, because the nonverbal behavior and affect of the patient can be observed and compared to reported information. It is important to maintain a connection with the patient during this time through eye contact, facial expression, and body language. This not only implies respect and support but also keeps the information coming because the patient can see that it is being received in a thoughtful manner.

At the end of the evaluation the psychiatrist should spend some time to debrief and to thank the interpreter. Providing information about the patient's story or about a dynamic or diagnostic issue will help the interpreter's education and will provide empathy training for future work.

Community Outreach

One of the major issues in cross-cultural psychiatry is to establish links and credibility with the community so that patients can be identified and can feel comfortable coming for treatment. This involves an active, sensitive outreach program. Our counselors, chosen partly because of their acceptance by their own ethnic community, have the role of conducting outreach. However, the best outreach in our experience has been through our patients who have improved and have told others about the program. Self-referrals are the most common referrals in an established program.

It does not start that way, and at the beginning the counselors need to contact community leaders—often religious personnel or elders—to explain the program. This effort may not produce referrals, but it reduces fear and resistance in the community. Often the psychiatrist goes with the counselor on outreach visits to provide information, but also to be informally evaluated by the community ("Is he nice?" "Can he be trusted?"). The informality serves both purposes. Community leaders often can give information about problems that they perceive and that need addressing. Family physicians, nurses, and social workers often know of patients who need treatment and make referrals. Some of those patients are very disturbed, psychotic, and combative. The treatment of psychotic patients may be helpful because the results are often quite dramatic and visible to the community.

Case 2: A Community Contact

The Vietnamese mental health counselor, Mr. Tran, who had been partnering with Dr. Smith for 15 years, one day reported that the pastor of the main Vietnamese Catholic church had recently been transferred to a new diocese. Mr. Tran suggested that Dr. Smith should pay a visit to the new pastor, who was now overseeing the ministry to a congregation of more than 2,000 Vietnamese Catholic followers. Dr. Smith set aside a whole afternoon one day and drove to the church as arranged. On his arrival, Mr. Tran was already waiting for Dr. Smith and quickly escorted him into the church office. He first showed Dr. Smith around and then introduced him to the half-dozen workers there. Fifteen minutes into the chitchat, Dr. Smith was informed that the priest was ready to receive him. Dr. Smith presented his business card to the pastor, who greeted him in an inner office. After the exchanging of formalities, the priest asked Dr. Smith to tell him about his work and, in particular, the area relating to the Vietnamese immigrants and refugees. They went on to discuss their individual viewpoints about the needs in the community and how it would be affected by the local political environment. The meeting lasted no more than half an hour, and they parted. The priest walked Dr. Smith out to the parking lot, and, as they shook hands to part, the priest told Dr. Smith that he welcomed a program that could serve his community and especially the people in his congregation. A day later, Mr. Tran was in Dr. Smith's office and reported with a big smile that the meeting had gone well and that the church would continue to support their services.

Sometimes conducting outreach for a program or a service involves targeting a key player or group in the community of the intended patient population. In this case, the priest happened to be an influential figure, not just in the ethnic Catholic Church but also within the general community. Good will from such people can go a long way.

To maintain credibility it is important to reduce barriers to treatment. Therefore, our service has no acceptance criteria. We take all patients referred and evaluate and treat them as soon as possible (within 1 week). Receiving rapid and effective service by a psychiatrist is a unique experience for most patients.

The Process of Outpatient Work

The Initial Encounter

As described above, both the psychiatrist and the patient come with personal and cultural histories, which make the initial encounter a challenge. However, neither is stuck in his or her own prejudices and can change as the interaction takes place throughout the interview. There are also positive aspects that promote the process toward a good outcome. The patient is in distress and pain and wants help, and the psychiatrist is qualified to provide it. With the right approach, therapeutic beginnings can occur, treatment can start, the patient can get some relief, and the doctor can feel satisfaction in doing a difficult job well. The major goal at the initial encounter is to reduce the patient's fears and concerns about being different, inferior, or unworthy. The approach by the psychiatrist should be friendly and respectful. It is often helpful to make small talk about the patient's ethnic group or place of origin (such as with a Cambodian, mentioning that Angkor Wat is certainly a beautiful monument; with a Bosnian, saying that Bosnia has been a tragic area of the world; or with a Chinese, commenting about the many excellent foods that originated there). This helps reduce tension and provides indirectness and a sense of safety. This contrasts with the blunt approach: "What kind of problem are you having?"

Case 3: Breaking the Ice

Mr. Savovich, a 54-year-old Bosnian man, had seen his primary care provider for a number of months for complaints of aches and pains in his back and joints. Symptoms did not improve with multiple changes of commonly used analgesics. He was then referred for possible depression. When Mr. Savovich finally showed up after missing two initial appointments, he was quite upset about being seen at a mental health clinic and raised doubt about the need to see yet another doctor for his pain problems. Sensing the resistance from the patient, Dr. Lee informed Mr. Savovich through the Bosnian counselor that he had been referred because of the clinic's reputation for helping people like himself, newly arrived in America from Bosnia. Dr. Lee told him that the clinic would not only deal with his medical concerns but would also help him deal with problems in life arising from living in a new country. Mr. Savovich began telling Dr. Lee his need to find a job so that he could support his family and to obtain a safe place to live so that his wife did not need to lock their four children indoors all the time. The counselor and Dr. Lee spent the rest of the hour talking with Mr. Savovich about his concerns in life and how those problems were affecting the well-being of his mind. Dr. Lee sent him home with the same pain medication he had received from his general physician along with an antidepressant to ease his restless mind and to help him sleep better at night. Dr. Lee also promised that he and the Bosnian counselor would help him to find solutions to at least some of his life problems. Mr. Savovich then returned to the mental health clinic regularly over the subsequent 10 months and went back to the primary care clinic only once for other complaints.

Patients coming to America from sociopolitically unstable environments elsewhere face great challenges in the resettlement process. What might often be considered mundane problems in life can be overwhelming to these new settlers. In the evaluation of the medical and mental condition of these patients, one needs to assess and be ready to offer answers to these stress-provoking life problems.

Acknowledgment of the Presenting Problems

The next step is for the psychiatrist to provide information that he or she already knows about the patient, acknowledging the physical symptoms: "I understand you had backaches and difficulty sleeping; do I have it right? Tell me about your pain." Taking these symptoms seriously and asking about them in detail establishes credibility and a sense of further safety. The presence or absence of more psychologically based symptoms—appetite, sleep, or concentration problems; anxiety, irritability—can be determined during the next phase of interviewing. Next the psychiatrist should approach the patient's subjective feelings and the phenomenology and the social effect of the symptoms: "How have you been feeling? How does it feel when you have these symptoms?" This provides for an evaluation of the patient's ability or willingness to express the events in psychological terms. Quite a sophisticated psychological understanding is often provided regarding conflicts, loss, and trauma. This has been seen in all ethnic groups regardless of education. The social aspects are often revealing—asking "How is your family reacting to your pain?" can open up a discussion of perceived support, neglect, or hostility.

Obtaining a Thorough History

The importance of a thorough social and developmental history cannot be emphasized enough. Knowledge of the patient's early life experiences, relationships with family members, exposure to conflicts or violence, education, work history, and (if applicable) immigration status helps to put the patient's life in context. If a person is in the country illegally, this needs to be handled delicately but with confidentiality assured. Current marital status, number of children, living situations, and income provide an understanding of the patient's immediate social situation. A medical history—especially concerning diabetes and hypertension—needs to be obtained, and what other medicines the patient may have been prescribed needs to be determined. The problem of drug interactions and the patient's confusion should be kept in mind. Alcohol and drug abuse history, as well as illegal acts, should be asked about.

The Mental Status Examination

The mental status examination is a complicated process, and the process of interviewing—observing behavior and the ability for attention and insight—will reveal much, but when clinically indicated, orientation and 3-minute recall are useful parts of the evaluation. Proverbs, even in culturally specific expressions, and questions about judgment have been less useful. The ability to abstract and evaluate the subtleties of interactions is best evaluated in an actual social setting rather than by interviewing. Baseline measurement of blood pressure is often useful because many medicines modulate blood pressure. Also, in our clinics for immigrants, the prevalence of hypertension is about 40%. An added benefit of checking blood pressure is that it allows the physician's role to be fulfilled and often puts the patients more at ease.

Case 4: Cognition Examination of an Ethnic Minority Patient

Mrs. Nguyen, a 64-year-old Vietnamese widow, was evaluated for a complaint of being very forgetful for the past 2 years. She grew up in the rural area of central Vietnam and received no formal education. As an adult, Mrs. Nguyen was making a living as a vendor in the village market. Her children brought her over from Vietnam 4 years ago. She has not been able to find work because of her inability to learn how to use public transportation. During the cognition examination, Mrs. Nguyen was able to tell the day, date, month, and year. She was unable to comprehend, and thus was unable to perform, the serial 7s or 3s reduction tests. She was given a handful of coins (quarters, dimes, and nickels), but she was not able to add up the amount or to hand over the correct amount as instructed. She was unable to count forward or backward from a certain number to a stated end point. She was shown three objects for memorization but could not recall them after a 2-minute span. After being told that she had been back to Vietnam twice since coming here, the clinician asked her about the route and the time it took to return to Saigon, but she could not remember enough to answer the questions. On the basis of this interview and other available information, Mrs. Nguyen was judged as having mental impairment involving multiple cognitive deficits.

The traditional testing methods that are useful with mainstream patients may not work with patients of different cultural backgrounds. The clinician needs to be innovative in coming up with tests for a patient from another culture.

Providing a Formulation

Before summing up and negotiating a plan, it is wise to ask if there is anything the patient would like to know. If the patient feels safe, he or she often asks, "Am I crazy?"; "Will I get well?"; or "Can you help me?" This provides good information for developing a formulation that the patient can understand, and the summarization should give the patient a model of symptom development that fits his or her understanding. For example, to a Middle Eastern patient who developed psychotic symptoms after an assault: "You are a strong person but you have been attacked, which caused you to worry and feel sad. The more you worry, the more tired your body has become, and your mind has become tired. You begin to imagine things, and lately it's been difficult to know what's true and what's not true."

Before discussing a treatment plan, it is good to recount the symptoms gathered in the interview—sadness, pain, poor sleep, confused thoughts, anger, low attention, and so forth—and to ask the patient which symptoms are the most important to treat. Use of the patient's major symptoms will correspond—partly at least—with the DSM-IV-TR diagnosis, such as depression, psychosis, or posttraumatic stress disorder. One can prescribe medicine that not only helps the specific disorder but treats the complaints and symptoms of the patient as well.

Discussing the Treatment Plan

In addition to the medication regimen, the treatment plan should include a discussion of the frequency of visits and the major topics to be discussed. The issue of cross-cultural psychotherapy is discussed in Chapter 11 (Culture and Psychotherapy). It is particularly important to educate the patient about his or her disorder; discussion of the course and the effects of treatment helps allay fears of being unique or untreatable. Many psychiatric disorders are chronic, and the need for continued treatment or maintenance is indicated. Patients often assume that, as in somatic medicine, a brief course of treatment (such as an antibiotic) will cure the problem. More appropriate comparisons would be with hypertension and diabetes, which provide models of long-term treatment.

Case 5: Concluding the Evaluation

Mr. Vang, a married 34-year-old Hmong father of four, was referred for evaluation and treatment. He and his family had moved from central California to Portland, Oregon, about 2 years previously. Due to English language problems he was unable to acquire stable employment. At the time, the family was relying on a small cash grant from the Aid to Families With Dependent Children program, which did not leave enough money for food after the rent was paid on a two-bedroom apartment. His general physician referred Mr. Vang after treating his chronic headaches for several months without improvement.

In the course of the evaluation, Mr. Vang presented signs and symptoms of depression, including difficulty falling asleep, early awakening, losing weight due to a lack of appetite, fatigue, irritation, inability to focus, a sense of worthlessness, and an obvious sad affect. He also expressed passive suicidal ideation and vague homicidal thoughts. He was obsessed with the need to get a job.

At the end of the session, the psychiatrist, with the help of the Hmong counselor, concluded the meeting by promising Mr. Vang that he would be referred to the county job assistance program for training and placement in one of the numerous manual jobs available around the city. The doctor also told him that due to the extreme stress in his life, his mind and body had become dysfunctional, and this had caused him to experience so many aches and pains in his body, to be so unhappy, and to worry about everything. The doctor told Mr. Vang to take the medications because they should help him to sleep better and worry less and would likely reduce the pain. The doctor also made it plain to him that he was not going to tell others that Mr. Vang wanted to kill himself because this would only cause the authorities to take him to the hospital and keep him there. The doctor also told Mr. Vang that he should not think about doing bad things to the children, such as killing them before committing suicide so that they would not need to suffer after his death.

The doctor told Mr. Vang that any such thoughts would cause him to lose his children to the authorities. Mr. Vang was encouraged to contact his counselor any time that he had such troubling thoughts. Mr. Vang reassured the team that he would not harm himself and promised to return for his appointment.

At the conclusion of an evaluation, an attempt should be made to explain to the patient the reason for the suffering. The clinician should outline a treatment that is aimed at resolving the patient's presenting symptoms and problems and is congruent with the patient's views of his or her distress and illness. Issues of dangerousness should always be addressed in a clear and unambiguous manner.

Of course, if history indicates a physical disorder, direct treatment or referral to a general physician is indicated. If one feels comfortable treating essential hypertension or simple infections or making a diagnosis of diabetes or anemia, this can be done at the initial session. For many patients who do not have primary care medical coverage, such interventions are very much appreciated. One of us advocates closing an initial interview with the following statement: "You have three things to do: keep your appointments, take your medicine, and don't kill yourself. Do you promise to do that?" The last imperative is not because suicide is a common event but rather to indicate that the psychiatrist is very interested in the patient's life and that life is valuable and must be sustained.

Suggestions for Clinical Practice

In dealing with patients cross-culturally, the strict professional boundaries instilled in American psychotherapy need to be blurred because human contact is an essential part of the relationship (Kinzie 1981).

1. *Be human* is the first rule—gentle, not too serious, warm, genuine, and competent.
2. *Be respectful.* Offer respect and caring to the patient.
3. *Take a full history,* including information about trauma and psychosis. Determine if these are within or outside the cultural bounds.
4. *Don't overrate culture.* The individual variations within cultures are much greater than the overall differences between cultures. Consider people as individuals first.
5. *Focus on symptom reduction.* Reducing symptoms is very important. Take physical complaints seriously; touching patients provides a direct experience with the patients and fulfills the physician's role.

6. *Don't try to solve every patient's problem.* Be modest in your goals and realistic about what can occur.
7. *Be clear with patients about the processes:* what happens in psychiatric treatment, medicine and its side effects, the frequency and duration of sessions.
8. *Help with appointments.* Take more responsibility for appointments: make sure the patients can get there, give help with logistical matters such as taxis and buses, and give reminders.
9. *Use an indirect approach often in therapy.* This blunts the unsettling directness of some of the more confrontational therapies. Talking in general terms about similar cases gives an indirect way of providing a model when not directly talking about the patient's problem.
10. *Accept appropriate comments and gifts,* and reveal some personal information. This often reduces the distance between the patient and the doctor.
11. *See the relatives* if they come with the patient's permission. Families are often involved and can be a source of great help, and their questions can be answered. In many groups strict confidentiality is not as important as it is in the predominant American culture, with its concern for autonomy.
12. *Be very clear about appointments,* but also be forgiving when they are not always kept.
13. *Be gentle with yourself.* When working in this field, mistakes—both serious and minor—will be made. Just as we should not be hard on patients and should encourage them to be more open and flexible, we should be that way with ourselves to sustain us through difficult times and also to be a model to patients on the flexibility needed in mental health.

References

American Psychiatric Association: Diagnostic and Statistical Manual of Mental Disorders, 4th Edition, Text Revision. Washington, DC, American Psychiatric Association, 2000

Boehnlein JK: Introduction: psychiatry and religion, in Psychiatry and Religion, the Convergence of Mind and Spirit. Edited by Boehnlein JK. Washington, DC, American Psychiatric Press, 2000, pp xv–xx

Boehnlein JK, Kinzie JD: Refugee trauma. Transcultural Psychiatric Research Review 32:223–252, 1995

Boehnlein JK, Kinzie JD, Leung PK: Countertransference in the treatment of torture survivors, in Caring for Victims of Torture. Edited by Jaranson JM, Popkin MK. Washington, DC, American Psychiatric Press, 1998, pp 173–184

Group for the Advancement of Psychiatry: Cultural Assessment in Clinical Psychiatry. Report No 145. Washington, DC, American Psychiatric Publishing, 2002

Kinzie JD: Evaluation and psychotherapy of Indochinese refugee patients. Am J Psychother 35:251–261, 1981

Kinzie JD: Cultural aspects of psychiatric treatment with Indochinese refugees. Am J Soc Psychiatry 5:47–53, 1985

Kinzie JD: The establishment of outpatient mental health services for Southeast Asian refugees, in Refugee Mental Health in Resettlement Countries. Edited by Williams CL, Westermeyer J. Washington, DC, Hemisphere Publishing Corporation, 1986, pp 217–230

Kinzie JD, Tran KA, Breckenridge A, et al: An Indochinese refugee psychiatric clinic: culturally accepted treatment approaches. Am J Psychiatry 137:1429–1432, 1980

Kinzie JD, Boehnlein JK, Leung PK, et al: The prevalence of posttraumatic stress disorder and its clinical significance among Southeast Asian refugees. Am J Psychiatry 147:913–917, 1990

Moffic HS, Kinzie JD: The history and future of cross-cultural psychiatric service. Community Ment Health J 32:581–592, 1996

Pomeroy C, Mitchell JE, Roerig J, et al: Medical Complications of Psychiatric Illness. Washington, DC, American Psychiatric Publishing, 2002

4

Culture and the Psychiatric Emergency Service

Louise Lettich, M.D.

Culture, Crisis, and Coping

Emergency psychiatry poses its own set of unique problems to be solved in the course of assessment and management. Because patients of diverse ethnic and cultural backgrounds visit the emergency department (ED), the practice of transcultural psychiatric care is common in this setting. A competent clinician needs to comprehend the nature of the stress encountered by the patient and the coping used by the patient to deal with the crisis—usually while working within time limits in urgent circumstances. On the basis of this evaluation, more culturally relevant care can be delivered in accordance with the patient's ethnic and cultural background. For individuals who travel to foreign lands, or for immigrants relocated to a new community, the ED is the most accessible part of the health care system. If new networks of crisis resolution have not yet been developed, or if these resources exist but have been exhausted, the ED is the next most logical source of assistance. In the interests of truly understanding and providing aid to a patient from another culture, particularly a very different culture, all efforts to make use of appropriate resources from the community should be expended. The language of the culture, as well as the language of the medical culture, needs to be communicated within the provider-patient relationship.

Cultural Challenges in Emergency Psychiatry

Immediate Care With Limited Information

It is in the nature of a psychiatric emergency service that a clinician needs to make a quick assessment and a tentative diagnosis for immediate care, even with limited medical information. This aspect of the problem becomes intensified if the patient is of a different ethnic, racial, or cultural background from the clinician. Beyond medical information, many psychiatric problems need to be understood on the basis of personal history, family situation, and social and community circumstances. Such crucial, nonmedical information is often difficult to obtain within a limited time for patients of different cultural backgrounds, particularly if there is a language barrier. Relying on a translator will more than double the time needed for an interview and other communication, and this will severely hinder the emergency work. Experienced and skillful language interpreters are invaluable for this reason. A clinician needs to be seasoned and experienced with these unique issues to make an accurate clinical judgment and to provide effective care in such emergency situations.

Common Psychiatric Emergencies

It is also in the nature of the psychiatric emergency service to deal with certain psychiatric disorders more than others—for example, acute psychoses, delirious states, suicide attempts, or violent behavior (Fauman 1995). However, beyond that, psychiatric problems present differently in different societies and in patients with various social and cultural backgrounds.

For instance, in contemporary Euro-American societies, many patients will be seen for substance abuse associated with either intoxication or withdrawal problems. Violent behavior associated with substance abuse is common (Bell et al. 1994). This in turn influences the types of psychiatric problems currently prevalent in these societies. Familiarity with the clinical manifestations of various kinds of substance abuse and treatment is necessary for clinicians in these settings. This may not necessarily be true in other societies, where substance abuse is less frequently observed. In contrast, dissociative and conversion disorders, formerly designated as hysterical neuroses, may be commonly encountered in emergency services in other societies. This is true in China (Luo and Zhou 1984), India (Dube 1970), and Saudi Arabia (Al-Habeeb et al. 1999) and among Ethiopian immigrants to Israel (Grisaru et al. 1997). Under such circumstances, properly distinguishing conversion disorders from organic conditions, including epilepsy, becomes an important clinical task.

In other words, in emergency clinics in different sociocultural settings, the clinician has to learn to deal with different kinds of psychiatric disorders. Similarly, in the same emergency room, the clinician may need to deal with different kinds of psychiatric emergency problems, depending on the ethnicities of the patients visiting the service

The Rapid Assessment

It is the art of emergency service to make proper diagnoses as soon as possible for immediate care. This requires reliance on the medical history and laboratory examination. To solicit the needed clinical information, it is important to lead the interview actively, coaching the patient and the family in providing relevant information in a limited time. Many patients and family members are not familiar with medical situations and are not experienced in presenting their problems. This is particularly true if the patients and families are from different social and cultural backgrounds and have a different concept of illness than a medically oriented one. For instance, the patient's family may present a story, based on certain beliefs and interpretations, that the patient panicked or became crazy after being frightened by thunder or possessed by an ancestor's spirit. A psychiatrist may be interested in whether the patient had taken any street drugs or had experienced a head injury before the onset of these psychotic symptoms. Working through the gap in knowledge and conceptual differences regarding the problem is a task that needs to be accomplished within a limited time—not to mention dealing with a language barrier, if one exists. When a patient has a language problem, it can pose a serious challenge in an emergency setting. The availability of culturally experienced professional translators becomes a crucial factor.

Adequate Involvement of Family Members

In many Western societies, medical practice focuses solely on the patient and tends not to immediately involve family members in the process of evaluation. Even if the patient is brought to the emergency clinic by his or her family, in the patient-focused medical system the family is often asked to sit outside in the waiting room while the clinician examines the patient. This pattern of medical practice may be acceptable in an outpatient service, but, in an emergency clinic it makes more sense to involve the family from the very beginning because there is limited time. Permitting the involvement of the family will certainly help the clinician obtain needed collateral information about the patient and will prompt the process of immediate evaluation and diagnosis. This is particularly true for patients of cultural backgrounds unfamiliar to the clinician. Such involvement will help the clinician verify reality and assess to what extent the patient's psychopathology deviates from that reality. The diagnosis of psychopathologies such as delusions (particularly of a religious nature) or other strange behaviors relies heavily on an understanding of the reality of the situation. Obtaining collateral information and validation from family members may be the only way to make such a determination. Allowing family members to participate from the beginning will reduce their tension and anxiety. It will also help the clinician assess whether the patient can be discharged from the ED and return home.

Minimizing Diagnostic Error

Many psychiatric symptoms and disorders are easily misdiagnosed even in ordinary clinical work, but more so in emergency situations. Cultural gaps and language problems often contribute to misdiagnoses. For instance, distinguishing between commonly shared cultural beliefs and delusions, assessing ordinary behavior versus abnormal behavior, and evaluating usual coping patterns in contrast to pathological reactions are all potential challenges for clinicians trying to make accurate diagnoses in emergency situations.

Assessment of suicide risk is commonly required for patients who are brought into the ED after overdosing or engaging in self-injuring behavior. Such assessment can be a challenge because in many cultures suicide is associated with shame, and people from such cultures may not easily reveal their suicidal ideation to others, including family members. Detailed collateral information from immediate family members or close friends about recent troubles encountered by the patient, and the circumstances in which the suspected suicidal behavior occurred, will be helpful to the clinician in making a proper assessment. A sensitive interview with the patient is crucial as well (see "Case 2: A Japanese Girl Drowning at a Beach," later in this chapter).

Recognizing the Potential for Cultural
Bias in Patient Disposition

A major function of the emergency psychiatrist is to decide whether to discharge the patient from the emergency department after a crisis intervention or to refer the patient for inpatient hospitalization. Race tends to play a significant role, not only in giving patients more serious diagnoses and shaping the quality of clinical care, but also in hospitalizing patients involuntarily (Kinkenberg and Calsyn 1997; Segal et al. 1996; Strakowski et al. 1995). It can be difficult to make proper clinical judgments without being biased by the racial backgrounds of the patients. This is particularly true in emergency circumstances when the clinician must make rapid decisions about management and disposition.

Cultural Considerations for Emergency Management

Dealing with Language Problems for Communication

Because of the need to obtain information for psychiatric assessment within a limited time frame, one of the most serious problems encountered in emergency work is a language difference between the patient and the clinician. The most desirable solution to overcoming language barriers is to rely on professional interpreters. However, being a suitable interpreter for proper translation requires professional knowledge, judgment, and experience beyond basic familiarity with the languages involved (see Chapter 1, Introduction: Culture and Psychiatry, on this subject).

Clinicians have often found themselves without translators, yet having to proceed with an emergency assessment. Even when there is no language barrier, observing the patient before initiation of verbal communication is recommended. Reassurance and the establishment of rapport still need to occur.

The clinician may be surprised to learn that a patient's inability to communicate adequately is not solely due to language issues but is also related to the psychopathology of the patient and the relationship and trust between the patient and the care deliverers. The following case illustrates this point.

Case 1: A Croatian Patient Who Did Not Want to Talk

Mr. Vladic, a 38-year-old man, was referred to a hospital in Honolulu by the merchant marines for an emergency department evaluation. The captain and other crew members on board had noted this individual to be "odd" and had kept a log of his behavior. Mr. Vladic was highly educated and worked as an engineer on the ship. However, he was also known to be a loner, and his baseline disposition was described as "morose." One night Mr. Vladic unexpectedly became agitated and combative. He revealed paranoid delusions that had been troubling him for weeks.

Mr. Vladic came to the ED with a translator, who was contracted by the shipping agent. The translator was able to assist with the interpretation of the package inserts for Mr. Vladic's medication. The translator also helped the paranoid patient develop a rapport with the psychiatrist. The female psychiatrist on duty, Dr. Sivich, happened to be American born with Croatian heritage that was apparent by her surname. The translator told Mr. Vladic, "Look, her family is from a town right up the road! We can talk to her—she's one of us." Previously, Mr. Vladic had been withholding and suspicious, not wanting to say a word, causing the emergency staff to think that he did not speak English at all.

However, surprisingly enough, after the translator's appeal, he spoke freely (in English) to Dr. Sivich about his paranoid ideations and his belief that there was a conspiracy to kill him among the crew members on board. Through the cooperative interview, the psychiatrist was also able to determine that Mr. Vladic had insight into his illness, had been compliant with his medication regimen, and recognized the need for further treatment with possibly stronger medication.

This case demonstrates that, besides language, the common ethnic background of the therapist greatly facilitated the interaction between the patient and the therapist. Thus, a trusting relationship developed between them, which certainly helped the clinical work in this emergency situation.

Case 2: A Japanese Girl Drowning at a Beach

Miss Yamamoto, a 20-year-old Japanese tourist visiting Hawaii, was drowning at the beach. Immediately rescued by a lifeguard, she recovered without significant injury. The lifeguard did not speak Japanese, and Miss Yamamoto did not comprehend English. Fearing that she might have tried to drown herself in a suicide attempt, the lifeguard called an ambulance, and Miss Yamamoto was sent to the emergency department for further evaluation. A Japanese-speaking psychiatrist was called for consultation. The psychiatrist learned from Miss Yamamoto that she had traveled with one of her female friends to Hawaii for a vacation. Even though she did not know how to swim, she had joined her friend, who knew how to swim, in the water. Seeing her friend standing in the ocean with seawater reaching only to her waist, Miss Yamamoto thought that the water was shallow, and she walked toward her friend. Unfortunately, the water between Miss Yamamoto and her friend was rather deep, and she suddenly found herself drowning. During the interview, Miss Yamamoto explained that the incident occurred purely by accident and that she was quite ashamed about creating an embarrassing scene. Miss Yamamoto was immediately released from the ED so that she could continue her vacation with her friend.

Rapidly Establishing Rapport for Care

Successful psychiatric work often depends on a good rapport between clinician and patient. The ability to establish trust is a crucial professional skill. This can be quite a challenge in emergency situations, when time is limited. Every means available should be used to reach this goal. These may include finding a suitable person to help with communication, gratifying the patient's basic needs at the moment, and assisting the patient in solving the immediate problems.

Although there is controversy about the role of food and meals in a psychiatric emergency setting, it is suggested that patients be offered food, particularly when there is a language barrier or a cross-cultural understanding problem. Offering food helps to establish rapport and reassure the patient that basic needs will be attended to. In some respects, food is an international language, a universal symbol of good intentions and benevolent care.

Experience tells us that offering drink, food, or a cigarette often reduces the patient's anxiety, either from the stress of the emergency situation or the added anxiety of being brought involuntarily into an emergency clinic. Drink or food can be a basic, concrete way to offer comfort when the patient and the clinician have difficulty relating to each other through language. Smoking is considered unhealthy and is prohibited in many public places, particularly hospitals; however, offering a cigarette is a social greeting still practiced in many societies, and it retains a symbolic meaning of good social intentions.

Case 3: An Italian Sailor in Acute Crisis Aboard Ship

Mr. Cupo, a married 32-year-old Italian man, was working as a merchant marine on a cargo vessel. While the ship was en route from Japan, Mr. Cupo had a disturbing conversation with his wife via cell phone. She told him that she was leaving him for her former boyfriend, who had been incarcerated for 10 years. She implied that she had married Mr. Cupo only because the other man was unavailable. They had two children together, ages 5 and 7, whom she had left with her mother.

Mr. Cupo became angry with the captain of the ship, who would not allow him to continue to call Italy. Apparently, the commander controlled overseas cell phone use by way of computer chips inserted in the phones. The men were permitted limited time to make contact with their families back home. Mr. Cupo initially assaulted the commander and then attempted suicide by overdosing on a headache remedy, leaving a note bidding his wife and children goodbye. Luckily, his shipmates found him in time. There was no doctor aboard, but through radio communication the crew obtained verbal instructions to sedate

Mr. Cupo with diazepam for the 10 days it would take to get to the nearest port, which was Honolulu.

In the ED, Mr. Cupo appeared quite distressed. He came with the radio operator from the ship, who spoke English fairly fluently. However, the radio operator, an older man, was clearly angry with Mr. Cupo and continually berated him in a loud, threatening tone. The radio operator admitted being annoyed that the crew had to go to so much trouble to ensure Mr. Cupo's safety. The radio operator was unable to assist with a satisfactory translation. He confided to the doctor, "I've told him he better behave, or else he will be in big trouble. Trust me, that's the way to manage this fellow."

The American psychiatric resident coming on duty happened to speak fluent Italian. The ship's officers were excused, and the resident sat with Mr. Cupo and talked at length. The patient's demeanor changed appreciably. His body posture was more relaxed, his tremulousness ceased, and he even began to smile at times. After his evaluation, Mr. Cupo asked for something to eat, preferably chocolate, and persisted in asking to smoke a cigarette. The resident in charge, after consulting with the supervisor, accommodated him on all counts. The resident also managed to obtain his mother-in-law's telephone number and assisted him in making telephone contact with his children.

All of these measures helped to reduce Mr. Cupo's anxieties and made it possible to complete the needed clinical evaluation, including a safety assessment, and make disposition plans back to Italy.

Clearly, language played a great role in resolving this emergency situation involving a foreigner in an emergency clinic. However, the clinician's understanding of the patient's cultural behavior, knowing how to connect with him in a crisis situation with adequate cultural empathy, and good clinical judgment in gratifying his unusual needs—giving him American chocolate and permitting him to smoke in the nonsmoking clinical setting—all contributed to the success in caring for this patient.

Making the Best Use of Available Opportunities for Assessment

The initial evaluation of the patient should ideally involve all available parties—including family members, friends, neighbors, or law enforcement personnel who bring the patient to the ED or accompany the patient for the emergency visit—because those persons may have witnessed changes in the patient's behavior and will be available to provide valuable collateral information to help the clinicians in making a diagnosis. This is true in any form of psychiatric service but is particularly true in the ED if the patient is in an acute crisis and may be unable to provide the needed clinical information. If there is a language problem, help from a suitable and experienced interpreter should be obtained from the very beginning of contact.

Group dynamics between the patient and his or her family members or the person who brought the patient into the emergency room need to be observed. The motivation for bringing the patient to the emergency clinic needs to be determined as soon as possible. Otherwise, suitable assessment and care will be hindered. For instance, in the case of the Italian sailor described earlier (see "Case 3: An Italian Sailor in Acute Crisis Aboard Ship"), the first translator omitted information in the course of the translation, and his intimidating manner further delayed efforts to obtain the patient's history. In addition, he appeared to agitate the patient. It is important to note when this occurs, and it is best to remove the agitating individual from the clinical setting. Sometimes these individuals require a separate psychiatric assessment.

The patient's family, spouse, or roommate may be acutely upset with the patient (e.g., the wife of an active alcoholic who has her own issues to cope with). They may also be a source of stress for the patient (e.g., a well-intentioned but intrusive family member who does not understand that the patient with schizophrenia is not lazy but is manifesting early symptoms of catatonia). Crisis intervention will be needed right away.

Determining the Relevance of Culture for Diagnosis

In general, competent clinical diagnosis relies on medical history, including personal and family information. In addition, culturally competent assessment requires cultural knowledge and empathy. Proper cultural insight, avoiding ignorance or mistakes, can lead to a culturally relevant diagnosis. It would be desirable for clinicians to have first-hand knowledge and experience of the cultures of all their patients. However, that is impossible to achieve. To make a correct diagnosis, the clinician needs to rely on the patient's family or friends or on medical staff members who have the same cultural background to provide cultural knowledge and an explanation of the patient's thoughts and behavior.

Determining how to properly incorporate cultural knowledge and culturally influenced mental status findings into the information required for clinical diagnosis is a major professional challenge. A note of caution is needed regarding two extremes: the tendency to ignore cultural input and the tendency to overinterpret cultural factors. The following two cases serve as examples of the need to consider cultural issues in clinical assessment.

Case 4: A Micronesian Man Who Shot Himself in the Head

Mr. Puchaka, a single, 31-year-old Micronesian man, presented himself to an emergency department several days after shooting himself in the head, right between the eyes. In the ED, Mr. Puchaka was alert and ambulatory, and he had sustained only entrance and exit wounds visible between his eyes and to the right cheek. He actually traveled from his home island to Hawaii solely for the purpose of obtaining antibiotics for the wounds, which had become infected. Only basic medical care is available in much of Micronesia, and it is not unusual for people to come from there to Honolulu for more complex care. However, the ED physician was alarmed by the case and requested a psychiatric consultation.

Mr. Puchaka admitted to feeling depressed about relationship troubles. His girlfriend had broken up with him many weeks before. He had been drinking heavily, and he impulsively took a .22-caliber gun and shot himself. At the time, his mother was in the kitchen and his brother was outside gardening. Mr. Puchaka had no memory of the events following the shooting, and he woke up in the hospital there. He shared with the psychiatric consultant that he had had a religious conversion. Because he didn't die, Mr. Puchaka was convinced that God had a plan for him. Mr. Puchaka's affect was bright, and he was no longer suicidal. The ED staff, experienced with trauma, noted the diagnosis on the ED computer board: "Self-inflicted gunshot wound" and were quite surprised to see the computer register the instruction "Discharge to home"!

In this case, it happened that the psychiatrist who performed the consultation had cultural experience in Micronesia, having lived there for several years in the past. He was familiar with the society and felt comfortable and confident making the appropriate assessment and disposition.

Case 5: A Filipino Man Who Believed That He Was Bewitched

Mr. Sangalang, a 50-year-old Filipino man, was brought to the emergency department by his family after they found him shooting his hunting gun into the air. An interview with Mr. Sangalang revealed that he did so to chase away the devil. He believed that he was cursed and bewitched by some of his enemies. He used his hunting gun to shoot the evil flying about in the air.

Mr. Sangalang's family and medical staff with Filipino backgrounds all admitted that it was not unusual for people in the Philippines to believe that a person could be bewitched by others and even possessed by an evil spirit. However, the psychiatrist noticed that the patient manifested other psychiatric symptoms as well. Mr. Sangalang said that his thoughts were often put there by a demon, that his behavior was controlled by an evil spirit, and that he was not acting according to his own will. Mr. Sangalang's thoughts were tangential and illogical, even when talking about a subject not related to the subject of being bewitched. His family members agreed with the clinician that Mr. Sangalang was mentally ill and in need of hospitalization for treatment.

The ability to distinguish between culturally observed beliefs, behaviors, or customs and culturally dystonic phenomena and pathological symptoms is an essential skill needed in transcultural psychiatric practice, including psychiatric emergency situations.

The Advantages of Crisis Intervention

Many ethnic minority patients and patients from foreign countries are not familiar with mental health services and will not feel comfortable utilizing the existing professional care system. They tend to shy away from mental health facilities even when follow-up treatment is recommended. Therefore, it is desirable to solve the problems as much as possible while the patient and family members are still in the emergency service. This is particularly true if the difficulties are related to psychological stress or interpersonal conflict, which will frequently respond to crisis intervention.

Cultural Considerations for Disposition

A psychiatric emergency service is not only a place to make diagnoses and provide crisis intervention but is also a place to channel the patient to resources for care and support after discharge. This is particularly true for patients and families who are unfamiliar with psychiatric and mental health facilities in the community, many of whom are ethnic minority group members and immigrants. Where to go to obtain needed financial aid and help for living, where to find a mental health clinic, how to make an appointment with a therapist for follow-up care, and so on, all seem like minor details but may be critical issues needed to help many patients. The types of health insurance and social welfare systems that are available and the types of groups or organizations that can provide support and care are information that the patient and the family need. Thus, adequate social work becomes an important part of emergency service.

One of the clinical challenges to be faced in the emergency department is the disposition of the patient. If psychiatric hospitalization is being considered, it is very important to consider the implications of such a step. Members of ethnic minority groups in particular often attach a strong stigma to mental disorders and fear being labeled as psychiatric patients after being admitted to a psychiatric ward. Adequate explanations and preparation are needed.

In summary, all good medical practices are needed in an emergency service, just as in medical practice in general, and are not omitted simply because it is an emergency situation. Patients and families—particularly from ethnic minority groups or foreign countries—who are unfamiliar with modern medical facilities and emergency services require additional explanations and extra attention.

Suggestions for Clinical Practice

1. *Establish a multidisciplinary network,* including trained interpreters and cultural experts. This is very helpful in meeting the needs of patients of various ethnic and cultural backgrounds on an emergency basis.
2. *Provide periodic inservice training in cultural competency* for emergency department staff. The goal is to increase cultural sensitivity, to acquire needed cultural knowledge for the population to be served, and to overcome the difficulties associated with language barriers.
3. *Involve all available parties,* including family members, friends, neighbors, or law enforcement officers, for collateral information. Maximizing this opportunity will facilitate an accurate assessment and proper diagnosis within the limited time available in the emergency setting.
4. *Extend the needed care to the patient's family or friends,* who are usually anxious and concerned about the patient, in the form of support, explanation, and recommendations. This kind of family-focused care is crucial for patients whose culture places a strong emphasis on the family.
5. *Be familiar* (beyond common psychiatric emergencies) with unique ethnic- and culture-related psychiatric disorders in order to minimize diagnostic errors.
6. *Be aware that extra flexibility may be required,* in addition to usual psychiatric emergency management, when treating patients and families of different ethnic and cultural backgrounds.
7. *Provide immediate onsite crisis intervention,* to the extent possible, to help the patient and family deal with the difficulties encountered. This is particularly important with ethnic minority patients or foreigners, who tend not to comply with recommendations for follow-up care.

8. *When making dispositions, consider cultural factors,* including the utilization of community resources. The cultural implications of psychiatric hospitalization should be assessed if such a disposition is considered.

References

Al-Habeeb TA, Abdulgani YI, Al-Ghamdi MS, et al: The sociodemographic and clinical pattern of hysteria in Saudi Arabia. Arab Journal of Psychiatry 10:99–109, 1999

Bell CC, Jenkins EJ, Kpo W, et al: Response of emergency rooms to victims of interpersonal violence. Hosp Community Psychiatry 45:142–146, 1994

Dube KC: A study of prevalence and biosocial variables in mental illness in a rural and an urban community in Uttar Pradesh, India. Acta Psychiatr Scand 46:327–359, 1970

Fauman BJ: Other psychiatric emergencies, in Comprehensive Textbook of Psychiatry, 6th Edition, Vol 2. Edited by Kaplan HI, Sadock BJ. Baltimore, MD, Williams & Wilkins, 1995, pp 1752–1765

Grisaru N, Budowski D, Witztum E: Possession by the "Zar" among Ethiopian immigrants to Israel: psychopathology or culture-bound syndrome? Psychopathology 30:223–233, 1997

Kinkenberg WD, Calsyn RJ: Race as a moderator of the prediction of receipt of aftercare and psychiatric hospitalization. Int J Soc Psychiatry 43:276–284, 1997

Luo HC, Zhou CS: Clinical analysis of 1,622 psychiatric emergency cases. Chinese Neuropsychiatric Journal 17:137–138, 1984

Segal SP, Bola JR, Watson MA: Race, quality of care, and antipsychotic prescribing practices in psychiatric emergency services. Psychiatr Serv 47:282–286, 1996

Strakowski SM, Lonczak HS, Sax KW, et al: The effects of race on diagnosis and disposition from a psychiatric emergency service. J Clin Psychiatry 56:101–107, 1995

5

Culture and Consultation-Liaison Psychiatry

Jon Streltzer, M.D.

The consultation-liaison psychiatrist not only diagnoses and treats psychopathology but also facilitates doctor-patient and nurse-patient relationships, resolves conflicts within the medical milieu, and generally tries to optimize medical management and the patient's psychological health. Cultural issues can be important in all these areas, as exemplified by research and case analyses. In addition, the consultation-liaison psychiatrist should be aware of the cultural aspects of medical illness and its treatment.

Psychiatric Conditions in the Medical Setting

Although all types of psychopathology are present in a medical setting, certain conditions, such as somatoform disorders, are more likely than others to be seen by the consultation-liaison psychiatrist. These conditions are much more likely to have cultural influences than, for example, delirium, another condition commonly seen by the consultation-liaison psychiatrist.

The following two cases demonstrate conversion reactions, in which psychological conflict leads to weakness and inability to walk. Conversion disorders are much less common in modern societies than when Sigmund Freud described them more than a century ago, but they may be more common in less developed societies. In these two cases the consulting psychiatrist is confronted with similar somatoform conditions, each of which has prominent, but different, cultural underpinnings.

Case 1: "Weak" Legs Prevent Completion of an Unpleasant Task

Mr. Faagai, a 32-year-old man from Western Samoa, developed a profound weakness of the legs, making it difficult for him to stand or walk most of the time. He was sponsored by his church to come to Hawaii for medical care that was unavailable in his country. He was evaluated by a neurosurgeon who donated his time. All tests were negative. The neurosurgeon told Mr. Faagai that nothing was wrong with him and insisted they walk around the ward together. This resulted in Mr. Faagai falling down and refusing to get up, claiming weakness. The neurosurgeon then called for psychiatric consultation.

The psychiatric consultant found that Mr. Faagai seemed surprisingly content with his condition. Mr. Faagai was a respected bible school teacher in Samoa, and he was able to teach class sitting down. Mr. Faagai indicated that he enjoyed violent movies. He laughed and said that the more violent they were, the more he liked them. The consultant asked Mr. Faagai about the use of physical punishment for students in Samoa. The patient acknowledged that indeed this was normal at his school. Mr. Faagai's wife indicated that before he became weak, he had been assigned the task of physically punishing any student sent to him for that purpose by any other teacher. This was because the principal of the school feared that all the other teachers had a tendency to be too violent. Mr. Faagai also told the consultant that he had two previous episodes of similar weakness. The first episode occurred when he was a teenager, after falling out of a tree. Mr. Faagai was relieved of chores and given special privileges for the following month. The second episode occurred in Australia one summer, when he did construction work to earn money to pursue his bible studies. He had to walk on high beams during the construction of a new building. He was quite frightened, but then his legs became weak, forcing him to quit the job. Recently, when his legs became weak again, he could no longer serve as the teacher who would administer physical punishment to the other students.

The consultant observed that the patient attempted to appear as if he enjoyed violence, which was a cultural expectation. In fact, however, it was very difficult for him to punish students. The consultant therefore prescribed a benign medication and told Mr. Faagai that he would get better. The consultant insisted, however, that Mr. Faagai had to be careful with regard to physical activities, and he would not be allowed to physically punish students, even if his strength returned. Mr. Faagai was given a note to take to the principal stating that, for medical reasons, Mr. Faagai could not serve that role. Mr. Faagai seemed quite happy with this, and his strength gradually came back. Soon he was able to walk to the airplane to return home.

Case 2: Shame Causing Severe Weakness After Childbirth

After an uncomplicated pregnancy and delivery of her first child, Miss Bautista, a 36-year-old single Filipino woman, was unable to get up and walk. Attempts to help her resulted in her immediate collapse to the floor. A neurological evaluation including imaging studies revealed no abnormalities, and the obstetrician was at a loss to explain her symptoms. Psychiatric consultation was requested. The consultant learned that Miss Bautista was a housekeeper for a wealthy Filipino couple who were spending several months in the United States. Miss Bautista was in regular contact with her family in the Philippines, but she had not revealed to them the fact that she had been pregnant.

A Filipino priest told the psychiatrist that the patient was feeling shame and that perhaps this led to her symptoms. When asked if she wanted to keep her baby, Miss Bautista said yes, but she became tearful. Indeed, when she was confronted about her response, Miss Bautista volunteered that the weakness in her legs was caused by the anguish in her heart for bearing an illegitimate child. Miss Bautista was encouraged to talk to her mother on the telephone, which she reluctantly did. Her mother was very supportive and understanding. The wealthy couple whom Miss Bautista worked for were also entirely accepting. They had been unable to have children themselves and were looking forward to having the baby live with them. Once Miss Bautista realized that her mother still accepted her and welcomed the baby, she became very happy, her symptoms cleared up, and she was able to walk normally.

Miss Bautista had been too ashamed to tell her mother of her pregnancy. After the baby's birth she could no longer hide or deny her situation. The loss of ability to walk was in the service of an attempt avoid the inevitable revelation. In Mr. Faagai's case, shame—resulting from his inability to comfortably comply with the principal's directive—may also have been involved. The presenting symptoms were similar in these two cases, but the cultural factors eliciting the shame reactions were strikingly different.

Culture and Medicine

In recent decades, medical practice has been influenced by what has been called the biopsychosocial approach, in which consideration in the care of patients is given not only to biological processes but also to social and psychological factors. In other words, treatment and prevention efforts are aimed at *illness*, a biopsychosocial conception of the patient's condition, rather than simply at *disease*, based on the older biomedical model. It is apparent that cultural issues must play an important part in this biopsychosocial approach. However, although the influence of culture on psychopathology is widely accepted, the influence of culture on general medical practice has received much less attention.

Culture may influence medical practice in many ways. The patient's cultural background contributes to his or her appreciation and presentation of symptoms, motivation for treatment, expectations of the physician, adjustment to illness, understanding of medical interventions, and compliance with them. The physician's cultural background contributes to his or her expectations of the patient and to the approach to patients who do not meet these expectations. Cultural factors influence the doctor-patient relationship, which is often a critical part of the healing process. In addition, treatment modes (such as inpatient or outpatient treatment), techniques (such as surgery or physical therapies), and values (such as the importance of prevention) can vary considerably in different societies and cultures.

Much of the literature that recognizes cultural differences in medicine emphasizes differences between the East and the West. In the United States, 95% of internists would inform patients with cancer of the diagnosis (Feldman et al. 1999). This contrasts with 0% of Chinese internists surveyed. These physicians were also surveyed with regard to patient preference regarding chemotherapy for advanced cancer. When family members' wishes conflicted with the patient's preference, Chinese internists were likely to follow the family's preferences rather than those of the patient 65% of the time, in contrast to U.S. internists, who would do so only 5% of the time.

It is noteworthy that in a United States survey published in 1961, most practitioners indicated they would not tell a dying patient of his cancer diagnosis (Oken 1961). This is similar to the current practice in China, Japan, and many other countries. Yet by 1979, U.S. physicians overwhelmingly indicated that they would inform the cancer patient of a terminal diagnosis (Novack et al. 1979). Parenthetically, however, there is significant evidence that U.S. physicians have difficulty providing such information despite their belief that they should do so.

A recent study compared the treatment of myocardial infarction patients in Japan and in the United States. Hospital stays were almost three times longer in Japan, although stays in coronary care units were identical at 3 days. Hospital costs were much lower in Japan despite the increased length of stay. In the United States a significant period of post-hospital rehabilitation is usual. In contrast, in Japan most of the rehabilitation takes place in the hospital, and the patient is much closer to returning to normal function at the time of discharge. In Japan the discharge decision is more flexible, and family members contribute a great deal to determining the discharge date (Muramatsu and Liang 1999).

Cultural Competence in Medicine

The need for cultural competence is gradually becoming recognized in medical practice. Several medical specialties in the United States have begun to emphasize this need, including family practice, internal medicine, obstetrics and gynecology, and orthopedics. In a 1998 survey, 58% of family-practice residency programs had at least an informal curriculum touching on cultural issues. This compares with 25% of programs that had such material in their curricula in 1985 (Culhane-Pera et al. 2000). As a result of concern about racism, proposed family-practice guidelines suggest that training in cultural issues will reduce the prevalence of unintentional racism (Ridley et al. 2000). In family practice, the ethnicity of women significantly influenced the diagnosis of emotional disorders (Kosch et al. 1998), and practitioners described discomfort in working with populations from different backgrounds, despite having sophisticated biopsychosocial approaches to practice (Bartz 1999). It has been noted with some concern in the pediatrics literature that in the United States there is far more racial and ethnic diversity in the child population than among pediatrician providers. This disparity is expected to increase substantially by 2025 (Stoddard et al. 2000).

The obstetrics and gynecology literature is beginning to emphasize the importance of culture. Estimates of pain during labor tend to reflect ethnic differences in care providers (Sheiner et al. 1999). Misunderstandings between doctor and patient are being recognized and considered important. Disagreements between doctor and patient regarding health status and effectiveness of treatment tend to occur mainly for illnesses with stress-related or culture-specific associations (Committee on Health Care for Underserved Women 1998). Similar trends in the literature are developing in some of the other medical specialties.

Medical Culture

In addition to cultural issues associated with patients and with staff, a medical culture exists that often influences the work of the consultation-liaison psychiatrist (Tirrell 2001). Effective communication with patients requires a bridging between the medical culture and the different cultural standpoint from which the patient perceives the world.

For example, there are differing role expectations for patients with acute and chronic illness. The acutely ill medical patient is expected to be a passive recipient of care. Diet, activity, bathroom privileges, and all activities of daily living are taken care of or prescribed by the doctor. In return, the patient is relieved of such responsibilities as work, child care, and even personal hygiene. The patient does not interfere with the doctor's treatment, the doctor is pleased with this, and the patient is content because he or she usually gets better.

With chronic illness, however, the situation is quite different. The patient is expected to become responsible for coping with and managing the illness, such as the diabetic who monitors glucose level and adjusts insulin level. Essentially the message is, "You are responsible for your illness: become educated about it and learn how to take care of it." Sometimes, however, the physician communicates to the chronically ill patient with a model of acute illness. The message from the physician becomes, "You are responsible for your own illness and activities, but at the same time you must do exactly as I say with regard to managing your illness." For some patients, this becomes a double-bind situation that leads to conflict, misunderstandings, and noncompliance (Alexander 1976). When this occurs, a consultation-liaison psychiatrist may be brought in. Clearly, cultural factors associated with the patient's background and with the physician's background can interact with the medical culture.

Case 3: A Battle for Control Between Doctor and Patient

Mr. Garam, a 50-year-old Eastern European man, was hospitalized after a series of transient ischemic attacks. He had received a diagnosis of insulin-dependent diabetes mellitus several years earlier. The attending neurologist requested psychiatric consultation, indicating that he thought the patient might have paranoid schizophrenia. He noted that the patient was doing well neurologically and would not need to be in the hospital much longer. The attending physician was concerned because Mr. Garam was constantly fighting with the nurses over his insulin injections. Mr. Garam was unhappy with the insulin regimen that had been ordered, and he was constantly trying to change it. The attending physician assumed the patient was paranoid and was fighting against needed medical care. The consultation-liaison psychiatrist obtained a history that the patient had emigrated to the United States many years before to escape a repressive government at home. Mr. Garam had been a physician in his native country but was unable to obtain a medical license in the United States. As a result, he obtained employment as a radiology technician. Mr. Garam was a proud man and a hard worker, dedicated to supporting his family. He had survived his tribulations by asserting himself and maintaining his independence, and he felt entirely capable of managing his diabetes well by himself. While Mr. Garam was hospitalized the attending physician wrote all orders for management of the patient's diabetes. Mr. Garam had no control and no input at all. By demanding changes in his insulin regimen, he engendered a great deal of conflict with the nursing staff. The consultation-liaison psychiatrist discovered that Mr. Garam's ideas about managing his diabetes were reasonable and were unlikely to result in a medical problem. Indeed, Mr. Garam had kept his diabetes under reasonable control for many years. The psychiatrist reassured the attending physician that the patient was not psychotic. He suggested that cultural factors were involved in the patient's need to maintain control and that perhaps, because there was no medical contraindication, the patient could be allowed to self-manage his diabetes. The attending physician accepted this explanation and was no longer concerned about Mr. Garam. There were no further problems.

There are many other areas where medical culture comes into play. One of these is the interpretation of somatization. This can be influenced by the underlying culture of the society, which may or may not be reflected in the medical culture. Thus, somatization may be an important form of communication to a patient, but to a doctor it may simply be a signal to search exhaustively for underlying disease. If the medical culture seems too alien to the patient, the patient may seek some sort of alternative healing. The following case demonstrates how culture influences medical care.

Case 4: A Quiet Man With High Blood Pressure

Mr. Cabuang, a 68-year-old first-generation Filipino man, was seen in a medical outpatient clinic in Hawaii, where he was being observed for high blood pressure. As was usually the case whenever he would be seen for a medical appointment, his wife was present with him. His high blood pressure had been discovered 18 months previously during a physical examination. He had initially been treated with a diuretic, but this had failed to control his blood pressure. He was then switched to other antihypertensive medication.

At follow-up visits his blood pressure fluctuated but generally remained high. The dose of the medication was doubled and then tripled and then quadrupled. The blood pressure had not really improved from the time he was first seen, however.

One day, the primary care physician asked the clinic consultation psychiatrist to interview the patient, suggesting that the case would be good for teaching interviewing skills to medical students. The consultant asked Mr. Cabuang how he was doing. As he always did, Mr. Cabuang responded, "Fine, doctor." The psychiatrist persisted and asked him if he had any problems at all. Mr. Cabuang responded, "No, doctor." The psychiatrist then told Mr. Cabuang that unfortunately his blood pressure still remained too high. Mr. Cabuang responded, "I am very sorry, doctor." The psychiatrist then asked Mr. Cabuang what medication he was taking. Mr. Cabuang responded, "Whatever I am prescribed, doctor." The consultation-liaison psychiatrist then became suspicious, and he asked Mrs. Cabuang, who had been sitting silently, whether her husband was taking his blood pressure medication. She indicated that she did not think so. The psychiatrist then asked Mr. Cabuang at what specific times he took the medication during the day. Mr. Cabuang responded, "I don't know, doctor." The psychiatrist then asked Mr. Cabuang if perhaps sometimes he did not take the medication, and he responded, "Yes, doctor."

Through persistent questioning it was finally determined that this man never took his medication. On each medical visit Mr. Cabuang always seemed cooperative, and his medication was constantly adjusted and increased, but it made no difference because he never took the medication at all. Actually, Mr. Cabuang had taken one pill the first time it was prescribed. He then felt lightheaded and dizzy, which he attributed to the medication, and never took it again. Mr. Cabuang did not understand the medication, nor did he believe in it. Therefore, he did not want to take it. On the other hand, because of his cultural background, the patient needed to respect the authority and the status of the physician. He needed to try to please the physician at all times, and certainly could not contradict the physician.

Because Mr. Cabuang seemed so cooperative, his doctor assumed the patient was compliant. He therefore wrongly assumed that the medications were always being taken as prescribed. Direct questioning about Mr. Cabuang's knowledge of the medication and about the way in which it was taken uncovered the truth. Questioning about the meaning of the medication to the patient might have revealed even more.

This case demonstrates two competing value systems. From the patient's perspective, he must not only respect but also placate authority, to the extent that complete candor is not appropriate. He must please the physician and act like a good patient. He seeks approval from the physician and feels obligated to respond in ways that he believes the physician wants. On the other hand, when it comes to actually taking the physician's medication, he feels free to make his own judgment, based on his own culturally influenced beliefs. Thus, he sees the physician as providing an *option* for treatment, which he will choose for himself. He does not believe it is necessary for the physician to know if he actually agrees with the physician and takes the medication. Their relationship is not one of a partnership in his care. The physician is an authority of higher social status and must be treated with deference. Compliance is a different issue. The authority of the physician does not mean he knows the correct diagnosis or treatment, and the patient feels free to make his own judgment in that regard. The physician's attitude is a critical variable in this transaction. If he mechanistically gives his prescription without showing interest in the specific understanding and illness beliefs of the patient, then the patient's true responses are more easily hidden within the doctor-patient transactions.

Cultural Competence in Pain Management

Patients with pain are commonly seen by consultation-liaison psychiatrists. Cultural factors have been recognized as significant determinants of patients' expressions of pain (Streltzer 1997). For example, the relationship of low back pain to physical findings explaining the pain and to psychosocial dysfunction varies substantially by country (Sanders et al. 1992). Some of this variation may be directly related to culture, and some of it may be related to the medical care system, including the presence of entitlements for disability. Historically, the article by Zborowski (1952) a half century ago perhaps remains the most well-known demonstration that culture can influence pain. Although no data were presented, observations of different ethnic groups revealed substantially different responses to painful medical conditions. It seems clear that culture influences the experience of pain, but precisely how and in what context have been quite difficult to determine.

An example of culture influencing pain management was the case of an Italian American postoperative patient who became emotional and verbal about his pain. His Chinese American doctor was distressed by this behavior, reduced the dose of pain medication, and asked for psychiatric consultation. The psychiatric consultant recommended higher doses of pain medication and discussed cultural issues to explain the patient's behavior, which satisfied the surgeon.

In recent years, opposite tendencies have been more likely to appear. A quiet, stoic, Asian patient did not complain of pain following surgery. The surgeon misinterpreted this as depression and anxiety and treated the patient vigorously with pain medication and benzodiazepines. The patient became delirious.

Looking back, issues in the larger society have been paralleled by changes in pain management approach, at least in the United States. In the past, fears of drug addiction led to general undertreatment of pain in all ethnic groups. Perhaps in response, dramatic changes in pain management approaches led to great improvements in the treatment of acute and terminal pain, but management of chronic pain has become increasingly problematic. As a result, consultation-liaison psychiatrists are increasingly involved in pain management (Streltzer 1994). Referring physicians request help in sorting out the psychological components of pain complaints, and they fear addiction problems. The importance of the consulting psychiatrist to overall pain management has been recognized by the American College of Graduate Medical Education, which now (since 2000) approves subspecialty certification for psychiatrists in the multidisciplinary specialty of pain medicine.

New technologies have led to improved surgical and nonsurgical methods to combat pain. Because pain correlates poorly with anatomical pathology, and because contextual factors are so influential, serious controversies have arisen with regard to diagnosis (e.g., fibromyalgia, reflex sympathetic dystrophy), surgical approaches, and indications for injectable steroids (Winfield 2000). In particular, a consensus has not emerged on the proper role of opioid analgesics in the treatment of chronic pain, and scientific studies have not clarified the issue because they have been subject to varying interpretations (McQuay 1999).

Today the consultation-liaison psychiatrist encounters a pain management culture that has developed in recent years with its own values, beliefs, and approaches to patients. This culture greatly increases the risk of opioid-related complications occurring in patients with chronic pain. These complications include misdiagnosis, prolongation and enhancement of pain, worsening social and occupational functioning, and increased medical morbidity and death.

The core values of this pain culture are consistent with the values of American and Western culture in general. Specifically, pain and suffering are not to be tolerated, and their alleviation is the primary goal of treatment. Furthermore, such treatment should follow a consumer model of medicine. That is, within reasonable bounds, the patient's choices should be followed. This is because patient autonomy is also a primary value.

A number of beliefs that go well beyond the scientific evidence have developed in conjunction with these values. The most critical belief is that opioids given over time are effective for chronic pain in a manner similar to that in which opioids given in the short term are effective for acute pain (Brown et al. 1996). This belief is quite controversial (Stein 1997). In fact, recent studies in both animals and humans reveal the development of an altered physiology with ongoing opioid intake that induces hyperalgesia, actually increasing pain sensitivity while inducing dependence on the drug (Vanderah et al. 2001).

Another such belief is that nonopioid analgesics are inadequate for anything beyond minor pain. This belief persists even though blind studies in patients who were not dependent on opioids do not reveal such prominent differences (Dula et al. 2001; Eisenberg et al. 1994). If one accepts this belief, then one also believes that the patient who fears the side effects of opioids and is reluctant to take them needs education to overcome this fear (Donner et al. 1998).

Another belief is that the patient's subjective report of pain is the gold standard for assessing pain. This subjective report has been promulgated as the "fifth vital sign." The risk involved in this belief is that somatizing patients whose complaints persist will be treated with ever-escalating doses of opioids or with increasingly invasive procedures.

This pain culture also includes the belief that there is a critical difference between dependence and addiction. In DSM-IV-TR (American Psychiatric Association 2000), *substance abuse* and *substance dependence* are defined, but the term *addiction* is not used. The new pain culture, however, interprets *dependence* as a natural aspect of opioid use that usually does not constitute a problem in achieving proper pain relief and does not interfere with function. *Addiction*, on the other hand, is defined as being associated with problem behaviors—such as lying, forging prescriptions, and buying and selling drugs—that are not proper in a doctor-patient relationship. The implication of this belief system is that if the doctor in good faith attempts to screen out addicts, perhaps by use of a signed contract regarding compliance, then he or she has eliminated the problems associated with opioid prescription.

Although this belief system accepts the presence of physical dependence, an often simultaneously held but somewhat contradictory belief is that the presence of ongoing pain generally prevents the development of tolerance. As proof, it is argued that many patients can go for long periods of time without escalating doses. Evidence for this phenomenon is only anecdotal, however, and tends to be limited to low-dose regimens. Moreover, there is no evidence that effective analgesia is maintained at level doses for long periods of time. There is a great deal of anecdotal evidence and some prospective evidence, however, that doses can escalate (e.g., Kumar et al. 2001) and pain may still remain and increase as a problem. In fact, a recent study demonstrated that ongoing inflammatory pain does not prevent induction of tolerance (Kissin et al. 2001). Nevertheless, within the new pain culture it is believed that if doses do escalate, it must mean that pain is increasing.

Interestingly, even clearly addictive behaviors can be discounted in this culture because of what has been termed *pseudoaddiction* (Collett 1998). This means the patient is acting like an addict (using medication faster than prescribed, obtaining pain medication from multiple sources) because more opioids are really needed to combat ongoing pain but are being withheld by the doctor.

Contrary to what one might imagine, patients with severe, persistent noncancer pain rarely have a clear-cut objective medical condition that accounts for the pain. More often, nothing is found that accounts for the extent of the pain. Persistent pain is more likely to follow minor injuries than major injuries, and the pain is likely to spread to other parts of the body from the initial source of injury (Streltzer et al. 2000). Because within the pain culture it is believed that pain complaints should be accepted at face value, it is postulated that secondary central processes leading to abnormal pain pathways develop in such individuals. The strongest evidence, however, suggests that such pathological pain pathways develop as a response to ongoing opioid intake (Celerier et al. 2001). Thus, long-term use of opioids may actually *increase* pain sensitivity.

What are the consequences of this medical pain culture? Narcotic pain pills are being prescribed in huge quantities. Diversion of prescription drugs into illegal channels has become a major problem, according to the National Institute on Drug Abuse. Deaths from overdoses of prescription medications have been highly publicized and have led to prosecutions of pain doctors. Workers' compensation costs for patients with chronic pain have skyrocketed.

What can be done about the dangers of this new pain culture? The existence of somatization must be recognized. Better understanding of the physiology and psychology associated with long-term use of opioids is needed. Above all, fear of addiction is not the proper argument to counter the overprescription of opioids. The issue is simply efficacy. The risks and benefits of ongoing opioid therapy must be evaluated based on different evidence than what is applicable to the treatment of acute pain.

Case 5: Twenty-five Years of Pain and Prescription Drug Dependence

Mrs. Flores, a Hispanic woman employed as a nurse, began using prescription narcotics for headaches when she was in her mid-20s. Gradually her use increased. She obtained medications from several physicians and also from friends. By the time she was in her late 30s, Mrs. Flores was dependent on 8–10 narcotic pain pills a day, and many physicians refused to prescribe for her despite her pleasant personality and attempts to convince the doctors of her special needs. Twice she went through inpatient detoxification, but each time she found a new doctor to give her prescriptions. When she was 45 years old, Mrs. Flores found a pain specialist who believed that her problems were due to undertreated pain. She was prescribed a combination of narcotic preparations. She always maximized the use of her "breakthrough" medications, and her total dose rose to very high levels. Twice Mrs. Flores was hospitalized, severely intoxicated with "accidental" overdoses while complaining of excruciating pain. On the third occasion of overdose, she died, at age 49. The prescribing physician strongly believed that Mrs. Flores suffered great pain and that the dose of opioids could be increased until the pain was relieved, because opioids have "no upper limit." He found Mrs. Flores likable and did not consider her an addict. He appreciated her praise for his caring approach.

Case 6: Opioids Worsening Pain

Mr. Moniz, a 55-year-old man of Portuguese ancestry, came from a family in which it was common to complain about health problems. In his case, he had been complaining of severe, unremitting back pain for at least 7 years. Five years previously, he had undergone a lumbar laminectomy and removal of a disk at L5–S1. This was ineffective at eliminating his pain, and 1 year later he had a second back operation with a fusion from L4 to S1. Mr. Moniz seemed to improve briefly after this second back operation, but then he steadily complained of worsening pain despite the absence of neurological abnormalities. He was unable to return to work, and his activities were quite limited due to pain.

For years his surgeon had prescribed codeine preparations, which had little effect on the pain. With no indication for further surgery, Mr. Moniz was referred to a pain management specialist.

The pain doctor immediately prescribed opioids at a higher dose. This seemed helpful at first, and the pain doctor was pleased. Soon pain complaints escalated, however; adjunctive medications were added, and the opioid dose gradually increased to very high levels. Mr. Moniz did not respond to several courses of physical therapy, acupuncture, and epidural injections. Because of increased irritability and moodiness, he underwent psychological counseling. Mr. Moniz appreciated this, but only minor improvement resulted. Finally, the pain doctor recommended implantation of an intrathecal morphine pump.

Psychiatric consultation was requested to rule out any psychiatric contraindication for such a device. The consultant found that Mr. Moniz was confused about the need for a morphine pump. He was accepting of it because his doctor told him it would be necessary to manage his pain. Mr. Moniz was not happy with his pain pills because they helped his pain only slightly and they made him moody and irritable, especially before it was time for the next dose. In fact, Mr. Moniz believed he was "hooked" on the medication because he felt so terrible if he tried to stop it or even to delay taking the medication. This had become extreme as his dose reached very high levels, and he believed that he would be stuck with this for the rest of his life. Mr. Moniz was willing to try the intrathecal morphine pump because his doctor had assured him that his pain pill would be available if needed for "breakthrough" pain.

The psychiatric consultant told Mr. Moniz that his physical examinations and his imaging studies were not that bad. The consultant suggested that he might have become "immune" to the pain pills, which were not allowing him to heal. Opioids had produced increased sensitivity to pain, and therefore the pump was not recommended. Mr. Moniz was happy about this formulation, which made sense to him. He agreed to new pain regimens and was gradually detoxified. The opioids were replaced with nonnarcotic analgesics. Mr. Moniz continued to complain of pain, but he became much more active and much less irritable. His wife was extremely pleased with the improvements she saw. Mr. Moniz explained this by saying that he still had a great deal of pain but he had decided not to let it take over his life.

Consistent with the new pain culture is the philosophy that if pain persists, treatment should escalate. Simultaneously, opioids should be used and the dose increased until comfort is reached. This philosophy was applied to Mr. Moniz, whose daughter called him a "typical, lovable, Portuguese hypochondriac." There were somatoform components to his pain, including a complaining personality style; nonphysiological abnormalities on physical examination; and the spreading of his pain complaints from the lower back to the hips, both legs, the upper back, and the head. Increasing doses of opioids made things worse rather than helping. Nevertheless, the pain doctor's response was to increase the dose further and further until an implantable morphine pump was considered. That solution would have been just as unlikely to relieve the pain as the escalating doses of oral medications had been and could have caused Mr. Moniz more complications. The psychiatric consultant used a different approach, taking into account the patient's personality, cultural factors, and the physiological risks of long-term opioid intake. The psychiatrist was careful to base his recommendations on the same value system as the pain doctor—that is, relief of pain and suffering. The psychiatrist was not concerned with "addiction." Once Mr. Moniz was maintained on nonopioid analgesics only, he continued to complain of pain when asked, but his functioning greatly improved.

Suggestions for Clinical Practice

1. *Consider culture in formulating the problem.* Sensitivity to culture is more complex in consultation-liaison psychiatry because of the medical setting. Cultural expectations of the sick role, the doctor-patient relationship, and treatment approaches must be taken into account when formulating the nature of the consultation problem and the resulting recommendations.

2. *Keep in mind the role of the family,* especially when dealing with chronic illnesses. Family members may be very helpful in understanding the important cultural issues in the medically ill.
3. *Be aware of medical evidence versus opinion.* A famous anecdote about medical education describes the first day of medical school, when students are told that 50% of what is taught will turn out to be wrong. Despite the current emphasis on evidence-based medicine, psychiatric consultation to help patients with their problems often involves more art than science. The consultation-liaison psychiatrist needs to keep up with medical practice enough to know when the science underlying medicine is clear-cut and when it is not. Medical cultures develop to fill gaps in medical science. Recognition of this allows greater effectiveness in planning solutions to consultation problems.
4. *Tailor interventions in the context of medical cultures.* When a medical culture is part of the overall dynamic, the consultation-liaison psychiatrist needs to tailor interventions to achieve the requisite result within the prevailing system of values. Even if beliefs need to be challenged, this is best done while supporting the core values.
5. *Be aware of the impact of pain culture on pain management.* Pain management has become prominent, and many treatment approaches are controversial. Beliefs about pain promise to undergo significant change in the future as clinical practice catches up with findings from basic science. The consultation-liaison psychiatrist should not be intimidated by the beliefs of the new pain culture and should assess the impact of this culture on the psychological processes that are so prevalent in chronic pain.

By the nature of his or her position the consultation-liaison psychiatrist has the opportunity to educate medical staff about cultural factors important in medical care. When the consultation-liaison psychiatrist discusses culture in the formulation of the problem, members of the medical staff may become more interested in and more open to psychosocial issues. By fostering cultural sensitivity, the consultation-liaison psychiatrist can increase sensitivity to psychosocial factors in general.

References

Alexander L: The double-bind theory and hemodialysis. Arch Gen Psychiatry 33:1353–1356, 1976

American Psychiatric Association: Diagnostic and Statistical Manual of Mental Disorders, 4th Edition, Text Revision. Washington, DC, American Psychiatric Association, 2000

Bartz R: Beyond the biopsychosocial model: new approaches to doctor-patient interactions. J Fam Pract 48:601–607, 1999

Brown RL, Fleming MF, Patterson JJ: Chronic opioid analgesic therapy for chronic low back pain. J Am Board Fam Pract 9:191–204, 1996

Celerier E, Laulin JP, Corcuff JB, et al: Progressive enhancement of delayed hyperalgesia induced by repeated heroin administration: a sensitization process. J Neurosci 21:4074–4080, 2001

Collett BJ: Opioid tolerance: the clinical perspective. Br J Anaesth 81:58–68, 1998

Committee on Health Care for Underserved Women. American College of Obstetricians and Gynecologists: ACOG committee opinion. Cultural competency in health care. Number 201, March 1998. Int J Gynaecol Obstet 62:96–99, 1998

Culhane-Pera KA, Like RC, Lebensohn-Chialvo P, et al: Multicultural curricula in family practice residencies. Fam Med 32:167–173, 2000

Donner B, Raber M, Zenz M, et al: Experiences with the prescription of opioids: a patient questionnaire. J Pain Symptom Manage 15:231–234, 1998

Dula DJ, Anderson R, Wood GC: A prospective study comparing i.m. ketorolac with i.m. meperidine in the treatment of acute biliary colic. J Emerg Med 20:121–124, 2001

Eisenberg E, Berkey CS, Carr DB, et al: Efficacy and safety of nonsteroidal anti-inflammatory drugs for cancer pain: a meta-analysis. J Clin Oncol 12:2756–2765, 1994

Feldman MD, Zhang J, Cummings SR: Chinese and U.S. internists adhere to different ethical standards. J Gen Intern Med 14:469–473, 1999

Kissin I, Bright CA, Bradley EL Jr: Can inflammatory pain prevent the development of acute tolerance to alfentanil? Anesth Analg 92:1296–1300, 2001

Kosch SG, Burg MA, Podikuju S: Patient ethnicity and diagnosis of emotional disorders in women. Fam Med 30:215–219, 1998

Kumar K, Kelly M, Pirlot T: Continuous intrathecal morphine treatment for chronic pain of nonmalignant etiology: long-term benefits and efficacy. Surg Neurol 55:79–86, 2001

McQuay HJ: How should we measure the outcome? in Opioid Sensitivity of Chronic Noncancer Pain. Edited by Kalso E, McQuay HJ, Wiesenfeld-Hallin Z. Seattle, WA, IASP Press, 1999, pp 371–383

Muramatsu N, Liang J: Hospital length of stay in the United States and Japan: a case study of myocardial infarction patients. Int J Health Serv 29:189–209, 1999

Novack DH, Plumer R, Smith RL, et al: Changes in physicians' attitudes toward telling the cancer patient. JAMA 241:897–900, 1979

Oken D: What to tell cancer patients: a study of medical attitudes. JAMA 175:1120–1128, 1961

Ridley CR, Chih DW, Olivera RJ: Training in cultural schemas: an antidote to unintentional racism in clinical practice. Am J Orthopsychiatry 70:65–72, 2000

Sanders SH, Brena SF, Spier CJ, et al: Chronic low back pain patients around the world: cross-cultural similarities and differences. Clin J Pain 8:317–323, 1992

Sheiner EK, Sheiner E, Shoham-Vardi I, et al: Ethnic differences influence care giver's estimates of pain during labour. Pain 81:299–305, 1999

Stein C: Opioid treatment of chronic nonmalignant pain. Anesth Analg 84:912–914, 1997

Stoddard JJ, Back MR, Brotherton SE: The respective racial and ethnic diversity of US pediatricians and American children. Pediatrics 105:27–31, 2000

Streltzer J: Consultation-liaison psychiatry 1980–90—the Hawaii experience, in Consultation-Liaison Psychiatry: 1990 and Beyond. Edited by Leigh H. New York, Plenum, 1994, pp 175–180

Streltzer J: Pain, in Culture and Psychopathology: A Guide to Clinical Assessment. Edited by Tseng WS, Streltzer J. New York, Brunner/Mazel, 1997, pp 87–100

Streltzer J, Eliashof BA, Kline AE, et al: Chronic pain disorder following physical injury. Psychosomatics 41:227–234, 2000

Tirrell SE: The cultural divide between medical providers and their patients: aligning two world views. Bioethics Forum 17:24–30, 2001

Vanderah TW, Suenaga NM, Ossipov MH, et al: Tonic descending facilitation from the rostral ventromedial medulla mediates opioid-induced abnormal pain and antinociceptive tolerance. J Neurosci 21:279–286, 2001

Winfield JB: Psychological determinants of fibromyalgia and related syndromes. Curr Rev Pain 4:276–286, 2000

Zborowski M: Cultural components in response to pain. J Soc Issues 8:16–30, 1952

6

Culture and Addiction Psychiatry

Joseph Westermeyer, M.D., M.P.H., Ph.D.

Introduction

Addiction as a Cultural Concept

The production, commerce, and use of psychoactive substances go deep into the prehistory of the human family. Archaeological evidence—as well as historical and anthropological evidence—from preliterate societies reveals that psychoactive substance use of some kind has been virtually universal across cultures. Most of the substances that are widely used today were available before written records, including alcohol, opium, cannabis, and various forms of stimulants (e.g., coca leaf, khat, kola nut, caffeine, and nicotine) (Westermeyer 1999).

Despite the availability of such substances, daily use to the point of disability was not widely reported in early historical treatises. Several factors probably accounted for this:

- Carbohydrate-containing plants for the preparation of alcohol were not abundant and farming them required considerable toil, so fermentation of carbohydrates into alcohol was limited to group, ceremonial, or ritual occasions.
- Daily intoxication was inconsistent with hard physical labor, hunting, and other survival tasks.

- Ecological niches as well as cultural values favored particular psychoactive substances, which then became the traditional intoxicant. Thus, the number of available psychoactive substances was limited.
- Cultures determined the person, place, and time of psychoactive use, and these dictates were reinforced by child raising, spiritual beliefs, and moral strictures within the society.

Anthropological evidence garnered from modern-day preliterate subsistence economies has shown that these societies can support addictive use of certain substances, such as opium, tobacco, and betel nut. Whether this also occurred in societies many centuries ago before the introduction of writing is less certain (Westermeyer 1992).

It seems likely that chronic alcohol inebriety, as contrasted with episodic intoxication, first appeared during the Neolithic period. Coincident with the preparation of more effective, finely made stone implements, agricultural innovations appeared. Out of these innovations arose towns and cities, regional commerce in foodstuffs (rather than simply in precious stones or shells), and a relatively more abundant food supply. Along with the cultivation of excess carbohydrate-containing crops, this combination of factors also permitted the emergence of salaried craftsmen, a priestly class, and a warrior-ruling class. Linguistic evidence from modern preliterate societies suggests that specific terms, such as *alcoholic* and *addict*, developed to label problematic alcohol and drug use.

The first two historical epidemics of substance abuse confirmed these addiction concepts. The Gin Epidemic was centered in England (but also involved rum and affected other countries of Europe). The Opium Epidemic affected Oriental Asia. Both epidemics began in the sixteenth century and increased dramatically in the seventeenth century, with anti-epidemic efforts continuing through the eighteenth to twentieth centuries (Fields and Tararin 1970; Rodin 1981).

Lay people, even if they are practicing addicts, understand the importance of labels (Murphy 1976). A few decades ago it was not unusual to encounter an alcohol-dependent patient who would summarize his status by remarking, "I'm just a common drunk, doc, not an alcoholic." In these cases the person was pleading for status as a normal person who episodically enjoyed drunkenness, instead of as a deviant, outcast alcoholic. In recent years the reduced stigmatization associated with the social status of "alcoholic" has lessened the aversion to accepting this label in the United States. The term *addict*, with its imputation of illicit drug use, still bears abundant social opprobrium.

Role of Culture as Etiology

Socialization consists of a society's education and training of its youth into the lifeways of the society. With regard to substance use, socialization involves role modeling supervision of the child by adults, with the goal of the child's acquiring knowledge, skill, and values in using psychoactive substances. Inadequate socialization occurs if the prescriptions and proscriptions regarding a substance are not taught to the developing child. To be effective, these aspects of culture must be taught early, beginning in childhood and continuing into adolescence. Some ethnic groups do an excellent job of socializing their children into appropriate prescriptions and proscriptions regarding substances (Graves 1967).

Norm conflict exists when ideal norms and behavioral norms differ in a culture. Ideal norms forbid use of a substance, whereas the actual behavioral norm may expect use as a normative behavior. The greater the gap between ideal and behavioral norms, the greater the presumed conflict. Norm conflicts occur when it is up to the individual rather than the entire society to decide between substance use and nonuse. It is this in-between area that most predisposes to substance abuse and dependence, especially for addictive substances such as alcohol and tobacco. From the public health perspective, societal prescription or proscription regarding use of a particular substance is better than lack of a societal stand (Hamer 1965).

Pathogenic use patterns can occur as a behavioral norm, especially in groups with norm conflict regarding substance use. For example, a society may idealize abstinence from a substance but then permit heavy binge use of the substance. A common pattern may involve alcohol use around the clock for an entire holiday, or a weekend, or over a 1- or 2-week vacation. This pattern is likely to lead to pathological use of alcohol in vulnerable persons in as many as half of adult males in some groups. Some behavioral scientists sanction this pattern as "normal" because it may be a behavioral norm or a statistical norm (i.e., most people do it) within the group. Clinicians or public health officials may view it as abnormal or pathogenic due to the high rate of death and disability occasioned by this pattern. In the latter instance, the argument revolves around the various definitions of *normal* and *abnormal* (e.g., ideal or behavior norm, statistical norm, health norm) rather than whether such a pattern is healthy or unhealthy (Caetano 1987).

Rapid, disruptive culture change can dispose a society to addiction. In such a context, *generational change* can lead to the replacement of traditional cottage-industry substances (e.g., locally grown tobacco, locally produced beer or wine) with industry-produced substances (e.g., manufactured cigarettes, imported beer or spirits). In some situations, young people may use substances that were completely unfamiliar to earlier generations. *Secular use* then replaces ritual or ceremonial use, individual choice replaces group decision making, and untried patterns replace patterns that had evolved over centuries. *Anomie,* the loss of a positive ethnic identity, is apt to occur in traditional peoples whose technological culture has been rapidly and extensively undermined by sudden influx of foreign influences. Rapid and fundamental changes in technological bases of a culture provoke tremendous changes in social organization, family relationships, cultural symbols, and other aspects of culture. Conquest by a foreign power with dramatically different values and mores can also precipitate cultural tumult. *Status conflict,* the discrepancy between a person's aspirations and his or her actual status in the community, can be a source of motivation, driving the individual to work or strive harder. An overwhelming degree of status conflict with no possible resolution can motivate one to accept the inherent risks of substance abuse or participation in the drug trade. *Disenfranchised* individuals or groups can assume substance abuse as a symbol and may play major roles in the drug trade (Kraus and Buffler 1979; Westermeyer 1999).

Technological changes can render a traditional psychoactive use pattern unsafe. Societies at risk in this fashion have typically accepted heavy, episodic intoxication at ceremonial times, during ritual occasions, or in certain types of work (e.g., mutual assistance in harvesting crops or building a home, public or corvée labor). The traditional pattern may have been acceptable because a heavy drinker riding home from a New Year celebration on an ox cart may be relatively safe and is unlikely to harm others. The same person riding a bicycle or a motorcycle or driving a car or truck poses a serious risk to harm self and others. Intoxicated mariners today risk the lives of hundreds of people (on a ferry boat) or an entire ecosystem (on an oil tanker). An airline pilot or a surgeon who is hung over from a bout of recent drinking can make small but lethal errors (Markides 1988; Stull 1972).

Migration may foster substance abuse in some groups. Refugees have been most widely studied with regard to their developing substance abuse in the new resettlement society. Some research suggests that this risk is not immediate (unless the migrant has already become dependent on substances before relocation) but rather tends to begin after several years in the new culture. Factors that complicate recovery in the migrant include acculturation failure, marginal socioeconomic status, lack of familiarity with the treatment and recovery in the new setting, and lack of treatment programs aimed at helping migrants (Westermeyer 1989a).

Role of Culture in Treatment

Treatment access requires first that treatment be *available* in the community. However, although a treatment program may be geographically available, it may not be *accessible* due to financial or cultural barriers. For example, hiring staff members from the affected community is a key feature in making treatment accessible. Finally, the patient must find the treatment staff and program *acceptable*. Toward this end, the staff can learn and perhaps employ the models of healing preferred by the patient population. The literature provides examples for developing culturally acceptable treatment and recovery plans (Husted et al. 1995; Westermeyer and Walker 1982; Zimberg 1974).

Cultural recovery consists of patient-focused behaviors that are conducive to sobriety, social responsibility, and good health. Examples of cultural recovery include the following:

- Regaining a positive, viable ethnic identity
- Reconstructing a functional social network composed of people committed to the patient's recovery
- Acquiring a religious or spiritual or moral commitment, recognizing one's commitment to goals and ideals beyond one's own self
- Undertaking recreation, hobbies, or pastimes that do not involve the use of psychoactive substances
- Establishing a responsible social role either in the recovering community or in the society at large or, ideally, in both of these settings

People in recovery generally return to their culture of origin (or ethnic group of origin). Old conflicts, aversions, and rejections related to the culture of origin create challenges during recovery. Infrequently, these conflicts may make recovery in the culture of origin impossible. Therefore, some people choose to recover in another culture or ethnic group besides their original one. Recovery as an adult in a foreign culture or ethnic group is not a simple, easy, or brief task because it requires the acquisition of new norms, values, customs, and sometimes even language (Westermeyer 1989b).

Recovery subcultures can foster recovery during its early stages. Typically these subcultures have their own jargon, values, customs, symbols, status markers, and social organization. A subculture composed of other recovering people, therapists, therapy groups, and self-help groups can guide the individual toward health and stability. These recovery subcultures can provide support as needed, can confront or challenge the recovering person according the situation, and can guide the person in avoiding dangerous situations that might precipitate a relapse. Culturally affiliated subcultures often provide a conceptual framework for recovery, which may involve "recovery work" guidelines and exercises or aphorisms that can become guideposts for recovery (Brady 1993).

Cultural reentry occurs when the recovering person, ensconced and functioning in the recovery subculture, begins efforts to reenter the larger society. This process may begin out of a desire for employment, education, or a family visit. The movement out of the recovery group into a new group or back into an old group involves risks. These risks include exposure to alcohol or drugs, loss or failure at a new enterprise, rejection by those who are biased against former alcoholics or addicts, and a myriad of other pitfalls. If the recovery subculture has done its work well, the recovering person should be prepared for this step. The recovery group can serve as a staging resource that can support and guide the individual beginning this journey (Godlaski et al. 1997).

Culture-Relevant Assessment and Diagnosis

To some extent, assessment and diagnosis need not vary greatly across cultures. For example, the elements of a substance use history remain fairly stable across groups. Some elements show both stability and diversity across cultures. The various elements of a medical history (e.g., review of symptoms, past medical history) should be present regardless of the patient's ethnicity. However, the clinician must be prepared to obtain dramatically different reports within these categories depending on the patient's ethnic and cultural background (Westermeyer 1987).

Substance Use History

What was your family's use of alcohol or drugs while you were growing up?

This query can disarm a defensive patient who is expecting to be cross-examined about the volume, dosage, or frequency of use. In addition, this information identifies the patient's early role models for substance use (or abstinence). This approach can also inform the clinician regarding the patient's socialization (or lack of socialization) into responsible substance use. The clinician should be alert to whether the patient's current substance use conforms with or diverges from the family pattern.

How and when did you first start using alcohol or drugs?

Again, this query avoids a judgmental approach while inviting the patient to consider his or her longitudinal use of substances. Did substance use begin in the context of the family, with close supervision by adults who monitored the amount and duration of use? Or did it begin in a peer environment marked by rapid, surreptitious use? Was the patient a child, an adolescent, or an adult when first beginning use? Culturally integrated socialization into substance use begins early, so a person without substance abuse problems is apt to have begun use while a child. Substance abusers typically begin substance use during adolescence or adulthood. There are exceptions, in which children in a chaotic household begin to mimic their parents' abuse of substances during childhood.

When did you first encounter problems associated with your substance use? What were the problems?

It typically takes some years from the onset of heavy or illicit substance use to the beginning of substance-related problems. This interim period varies with the type of substance, being longer on average with alcohol (8–12 years, depending on the group studied) and shorter with cocaine and opiates (typically around 3 years). Of course, there is considerable variation: some people develop problems within months, whereas others go decades before experiencing problems. As a general rule, psychosocial problems tend to begin earlier, often in association with very heavy use. Biomedical problems tend to begin later, usually in association with heavy but controlled use or episodic use. Again, the variation is considerable; a suicide attempt may occur after two decades of abuse, whereas a long bone fracture may occur after only months of substance abuse.

How has your substance of choice helped you function in your life?

Typically, substances helped the abuser function more effectively during early use. The ways in which substances can facilitate health and function in early stages are myriad. They include relief of insomnia, sadness, anger, racing thoughts, sexual dysfunction, social phobia, the gap between aspirations and accomplishments, anxiety or panic attacks, dysphoria associated with hallucinations or delusions, pain—the list includes virtually any symptom or malady. Over time the substance no longer relieves the problem as it did originally. For example, someone taking a substance to relieve premature ejaculation may eventually lose libido. Or a worker who takes a substance to relieve a simple phobia or social phobia on the job may no longer have a job. Nonetheless, discovering the rationale for use may facilitate recovery by pointing the way toward effective interventions during recovery. Examples include cognitive-behavioral therapy for an anxiety disorder, or medication for a chronic, recurrent mood disorder.

What has been your use of substances in the last 24 hours? The last week? The last month? The last year? Over your lifetime?

These specific questions call for specific answers. Several subgroups of patients respond with specific information. These subgroups include people who are not abusing substances; the substance abuser who wants help for his or her disorder; and the late-stage substance abuser who does not care what others think and is nondefensive about his or her use. All of these people are likely to provide relevant qualitative information (e.g., type of substance, route of administration) and quantitative information (e.g., dose, duration, frequency of use). The clinician simply needs to allow sufficient time for the patient to provide all the information requested. This can take seconds in the case of a nonabuser, up to 20 or 30 minutes in the case of a polysubstance abuser with a long history. Patients who are ambivalent about their use respond with a nonspecific answer, such as "I use about the same amount as my friends" or "I probably use the same amount as you do, doc." In some cases patients blatantly deny use even though their urine, blood, or breath tests are positive for alcohol or drugs. The latter type of response is highly associated with a substance use disorder.

Other Sources of Information

Generally, the patient is the most valid source of information. However, other sources of information can suggest a substance use disorder. These include all the various categories of data that clinicians employ. Examples include the following:

- *Review of systems:* hangover symptoms (e.g., headache, fatigue, nausea, vomiting, diarrhea)
- *Medical history:* increased prevalence of trauma (e.g., accidents, fights, rape), infectious diseases (e.g., lower respiratory illness, sexually transmitted infections, hepatitis)

- *Family history:* increased prevalence of parental loss during childhood, familial substance abuse or mood disorder
- *Social history:* declining socioeconomic status over time, underemployment or frequent job shifts; divorce associated with substance abuse; avocations that center on substance use
- *Examination:* evidence of physical complications (e.g., rhinophyma, enlarged tender liver, bruises and abrasions, spider nevi)
- *Laboratory data* (e.g., abnormal liver function tests, increased mean corpuscular volume of red blood cells)
- *Collateral sources* of information (e.g., from spouse, roommates, case managers)
- *Clinical course* (e.g., failure to respond to treatment, noncompliance)

Culture and ethnicity can affect all of these sources of information. For example, someone from a patriarchal family system may exclude maternal relatives from the family history reports, although maternal inheritance may rank as important as paternal inheritance. In some groups, family and friends readily provide input to a trusted clinician regarding a patient. In other groups, an individual may provide abundant information regarding him- or herself to a trusted clinician but may be reluctant to provide any information regarding other people.

Questionnaires and Rating Scales

Numerous questionnaires and rating scales can be used to screen for alcoholism and drug abuse. Most of these require only a few minutes to administer. Some require that the clinician pose questions to the patient. Others involve paper-and-pencil queries. Still others can involve computer-based algorithms, in which positive or negative responses determine subsequent questions (Davidson 1987).

Some of these scales have undergone cross-cultural assessment. For example, the Michigan Alcohol Screening Test (Selzer 1971) and its modification to include drug abuse (Westermeyer and Neider 1988) have performed well in many ethnic groups. A four-question interview format, the CAGE (Mayfield et al. 1974), has shown problems in use with diagnostic subgroups and could present problems across ethnic or cultural groups due to the nature of the questions. The CAGE questions are as follows:

- Cut down: Have you ever felt you should *cut down* on your drinking?
- Annoyed: Have people *annoyed* you by criticizing your drinking?

- Guilty: Have you ever felt *guilty* about your drinking?
- Eye-opener: Have you ever taken an *eye-opener* (a drink first thing in the morning) to steady your nerves or get rid of a hangover?

Diagnosis

At the margins of substance use disorders, differences can exist across cultures. For example, a decade ago some North American clinicians pushed for the inclusion in the *International Statistical Classification of Diseases and Related Health Problems,* Tenth Revision (ICD-10), of a V code indicating "pathogenic substance use" for heavy, pathogenic use that was not yet associated with identified problems. This recommendation was overruled, largely by clinicians from Europe. Likewise, the boundary between substance abuse and substance dependence has shifted over time. Despite these differences, application of diagnostic criteria has shown extremely high interrater reliability. This high diagnostic agreement has been true even when different diagnostic systems (with their diverse criteria) have been applied to the same group of patients (Westermeyer 1985).

Agreement between medical diagnoses and lay or folk diagnoses of alcoholism or drug addiction have been more uneven. At times the family or community may identify a substance problem when the clinician does not. The following cases provide examples.

Case 1: A Father Fears Son's Drinking

Dr. Smith, a European American physician, brought his eldest son, James, a 21-year-old college student, to the clinic alleging that James had become an alcoholic. Dr. Smith (and his family) belonged to an abstinence-oriented religion that proscribed any psychoactive substance use. During the previous year while away at college, James had consumed his first alcoholic beverage in the company of his peers. While at home over a vacation, he had gone out with friends and had consumed two alcoholic beverages. Queried by Dr. Smith about the night's activities, the son had admitted his moderate use of alcohol. This admission precipitated a crisis for Dr. Smith, who saw his son as initiating the "slippery slope" into alcoholism. Intervention consisted of individual sessions with the parents and with James to clarify the nature of the crisis as well as James's intentions regarding the family's highly valued religious affiliation. The therapist helped Dr. Smith accept that alcoholism was not present at the current time and was not inevitable in the future. In addition, in sessions with the father and son, the son came to appreciate his father's caring concern for him as he was beginning life on his own. Both James and his parents were doing well at the time of a 1-year follow-up.

Case 2: One Drink

Dr. Compton, a young female veterinarian, established a large-animal practice in a rural area of the South in which abstinence-oriented religion predominated. A member of the community reported her to the state board of veterinary medicine because she had been seen drinking one beer at the end of the day at the invitation of a family for whom she had worked during the afternoon. Thorough evaluation was entirely negative for substance abuse. Dr. Compton came to realize that she had broken a taboo in the local community. The board took no action in the case.

At the other end of the spectrum are cases in which the professional discerns a substance abuse diagnosis but the family does not, as in this case:

Case 3: Forty Years of Heavy Drinking

Mr. Cortez, a 56-year-old Hispanic, married, employed railroad engineer, was brought to the hospital with bleeding esophageal varices. Laboratory evaluation revealed elevated liver enzyme and bilirubin concentrations with decreased albumin level; antibody studies for hepatitis were negative. He had drunk about six beers each evening over the past 40 years, with greater intake on weekends and during vacations (12 beers or more). After a consultation, Mr. Cortez was informed of his alcohol abuse diagnosis and was referred for treatment. He refused treatment, despite the potential seriousness of his resuming alcohol use. His family (wife, two daughters, and son) would not consider initiating commitment, because they stated that Mr. Cortez could not be an alcoholic in view of his stable employment, his care and concern for his family, and the absence of fighting or troublemaking in the local community. This scenario repeated itself again a few months later, with a subsequent admission for esophageal bleeding. Mr. Cortez died of blood loss during his third esophageal hemorrhage before he could reach the hospital.

Normative Versus Deviant Versus Pathological Alcohol and Drug Use

The term *normative* can obfuscate discussion of substance use because it can refer to quite divergent concepts. It may denote a statistical norm (i.e., the type of substance use that most people engage in) or an ideal cultural norm (i.e., a mode of behavior that people are expected to follow but in fact may not follow). It can also relate to behaviors that are healthful or are considered normal as opposed to pathological or deviant. The latter meaning involves scientific concepts (e.g., sociological, psychological, psychiatric) regardless of social or behavioral norms.

Even among scientific meanings differences can exist, so a behavior may be socially deviant without necessarily being pathological from a health perspective (or vice versa). It is conceivable that a behavior may be socially conforming (e.g., participating in a weekend binge involving heavy drinking) and still be pathological, or at least pathogenic (i.e., capable of causing pathology, such as fights, car accidents, overdose, or withdrawal) (Jessor et al. 1968; Sutker et al. 1980; Westermeyer 1983).

Ceremonial Versus Secular Use

Socially sanctioned groups rather than individuals determine ceremonial drinking or drug use. Examples would include various Christian churches and the use of wine in a sacrament at religious celebrations, the drinking of wine within the extended family at Jewish Passover, or the consumption of peyote at rituals of the Native American Church. In these instances group traditions govern who may use the substance, in what doses, and over what period of time. Ordinarily, the user is protected when use occurs within a ceremonial context. This is not invariably the case, however; Catholic priests not socialized into alcohol use can become alcoholic as a result of exposure to ceremonial wine, or members of the Native American Church may abuse peyote. Such cases tend to be infrequent, however (Bergman 1971).

Secular use occurs outside of these institutional or ceremonial constraints. The individual or small peer group determines the occasion, amount, and duration of use. Traditional limits may not operate so effectively, even when ideal norms are known and often followed. Behavioral norms may deviate from these ideal norms, placing the user at risk for substance abuse. Cases of substance abuse usually arise from secular rather than ceremonial use of a substance.

Group Versus Individual Decisions and Control

From the information presented in the preceding section one might conclude that group control over substance use might be a key to healthful use of substances. However, this is not necessarily the case. Secret use within a peer group may be pathogenic. Such use may involve illicit drugs (e.g., cannabis, heroin) or illegal use (e.g., buying and consuming alcohol as a minor among peers). Use outside of a ceremonial setting also increases the risk associated with use.

Use restricted to a multigenerational family unit is ordinarily safe from a health perspective. Such use usually occurs in a festive circumstance, with eating and conviviality.

Between these two extremes lies the drinking or drug use context that is probably most widespread in many societies today: the controlled but secular use of substances within a family or friendship group. Examples might include a khat party in East Africa, opium served at a wedding in India, friends gathering at a tavern after work on Friday, or a couple having a weekend dinner accompanied by wine. In the vast majority of such instances, substance use appears to subserve social interaction that is healthy. Risk of addiction does exist in these settings. It often falls to friends and family members to identify the heavy or pathogenic user and to undertake a difficult intervention with the affected person. In other words, maintenance of healthful substance use in these settings inevitably involves monitoring not only of oneself but also of others in the group.

Substances may provide a major element for a group's existence. Examples include opium dens in Asia, cocaine houses in the United States, and tavern or cocktail lounge groups whose primary purpose is heavy substance use in a sheltered or protected setting. Such groups foster heavy, frequent substance use that often becomes unhealthy in time (Westermeyer 1999).

Pathogenic Factors Within a Culture

Cultural factors may also contribute to the risk of developing unhealthy use of alcohol or drugs. For example, a person not socialized into use of a substance within the family can develop substance abuse when exposed to the types of group use described above. A common American example is the person raised in an abstinence-oriented family who begins alcohol use while in college or military service.

Belonging to a culture or ethnic group that prizes abstinence while abiding substance use also poses a risk. In such groups, any use of the proscribed substance contains an element of social deviance for the individual. Examples include Irish and Scots peoples, some American Indian groups, and Muslim people raised to value abstinence. Although many such people can learn to use substances healthfully during adulthood, they do run special risks.

Role of Culture in Diagnosis of Addiction

Clinicians may encounter problems in diagnosing cases of addiction, in which the consequences hinge largely on illicit aspects (e.g., the high price of the substance leading to the commission of illegal acts, or trafficking in the substance as a means of obtaining the substance). Indeed, such consequences may be the only problems associated with use in some cases, especially among young people or those early in their substance use careers.

Laws Versus Cultural Traditions

At times laws run counter to accepted traditions. For example, use of peyote is against the law in most states in the United States, but peyote is a sacramental substance in the Native American Church. Most states now forbid the import or sale of khat, but many Somali and Ethiopian immigrants to the United States enjoy its use, especially if they are Muslim and thus forbidden to use alcohol. Many Southeast Asian refugees like having access to opium for use as a medicinal, a social lubricant, or a personal recreational drug. Over time, use of these proscribed substances tends to become associated with abuse in many if not all cases. For example, a study of khat use among African immigrants in London determined that there is a high rate of abuse (Griffiths 1999). Likewise, Southeast Asian refugees in the United States who use opium tend to acquire a cascade of social, financial, and health consequences from its use (Westermeyer et al. 1991).

Ethnic and Mainstream Similarities and Differences

A challenge posed to multiethnic societies lies in the differences among various ethnic groups with regard to substance use. For example, many religious groups in the United States do not accept the use of alcohol, tobacco, or caffeine—all of which are legal for adults to use. Thus, these groups do not socialize their young members into healthful use of these substances. From a societal perspective, this is not a problem unless the individual chooses to leave the ethnic enclave and join mainstream society. At that juncture, risk of substance abuse increases.

Likewise, many ethnic groups have a tradition of substance use that is not approved by the mainstream or majority society. Khat, opium, and peyote were mentioned above (Kennedy et al. 1980; Martin and Zweben 1993). Use of cannabis, heroin, and cocaine also varies greatly by ethnic group and geographic region, suggesting that group preferences are operating. At times, use of the substance may impersonate nationalistic feelings, such as with the manufacture and consumption of illicit alcoholic poteen by the Irish during their struggles against their English masters.

This variability in ethnic traditions poses serious problems in prevention for societies around the world, because most nations are multiethnic. On a national or state level, making laws for or against use of substances inevitably becomes a cultural exercise in which the majority usually rules. However, on a community level, the matter is more complex. For example, Native American communities racked by alcoholism have initiated grassroots programs to establish abstinence and prohibition as community norms. Some Muslim groups are establishing youth programs to guide adolescents and young adults away from use of alcohol (as well as away from other deviant or irresponsible behaviors) (Taylor 1987).

Drug/Alcohol Subcultures

Examples of drug and alcohol subcultures were mentioned earlier. These groups tend to involve finite numbers of people, many of whom know one another or at least recognize one another. The pathogenic aspects of such groups cannot be overstated. Nonetheless, these subcultural groups perform many functions for their members, many of whom have become alienated from or marginal within the majority society. These advantages include the opportunity to socialize and meet others, find out about jobs, hear the local news, eat, or obtain shelter (Dumont 1967; Weibel-Orlando 1985; Westermeyer 1974).

As subcultures, these groups depend on the mainstream or majority culture for their existence. Whether officially sanctioned cocktail lounges or illegal crack houses, their existence depends on the community in which they exist. To the extent that the community does not meet the needs of substance abusers, they will form into subcultural groups to meet their common needs. Local entrepreneurs (e.g., opium den or tavern or crack house proprietors) will identify the need and fill it.

Cultural Aspects of Addiction Treatment

The Intimate Social Network and Recovery

Most people have 20 to 30 members in their "intimate social network," which is composed of people whom they see regularly and who are emotionally significant to them. These people can generally be divided into four or five groups, such as the household group, important relatives, friends, co-workers, and those who share specific interests or activities (e.g., church, hobbies). Treatment of substance abuse can divide a patient's social network in half when he or she opts out of daily trips to a tavern or weekend activities that require drinking or drug use (Westermeyer and Neider 1988).

Clinicians thus help patients recover by assisting them in "social re-engineering" of their social networks. This step can hamper recovery, because most healthy people are fully committed to their social networks and cannot easily add new members. In addition, one tends to join the social networks of others through membership in a group, rather than as an individual.

Affiliation with new groups can occur through religious and ethnic affiliations. If the recovering person is alienated from previous affiliations, he or she may need to find new ones (e.g., joining a new religious group or affiliating with a nonethnic association). These group affiliations, whether old or new, perform a critical role in the patient's ultimate recovery (Red Horse 1982).

Course of Recovery in Titer Versus Binge Drinkers

Some ethnic groups, as well as individuals, are given to episodic or binge use of substances. Northern Europeans, northern Asians, and northern American Indian tribes tend to drink in this fashion. Rationales for heavy drinking consist of the weekend away from work, a vacation such as a hunting or fishing trip, or certain holidays such as New Year's Eve or St. Patrick's Day. Binge drinkers can often maintain longer periods of abstinence, over many months, without necessarily undergoing the recovery process that reduces their vulnerability to subsequent relapse. Ongoing monitoring, low-intensity treatment, and affiliation with self-help groups must continue over several years or a decade before sobriety can be well established (Robin et al. 1998).

Daily or titer users have more difficulty beginning even short periods of sobriety. Although sobriety looms more difficult in the short run, they tend to adjust more definitively to sobriety after several months or a few years. Relapse is always a risk but is probably a smaller risk after a few years compared with that of binge users.

Joining a Recovery Subculture

Like tavern or opium den subcultures, recovery subcultures can meet multiple needs. These include access to new friends with a similar lifestyle, information about jobs, role modeling for recreational activities that do not require or involve substance use, and other social functions. Many of these groups are spontaneous and informal and are composed of people who went through treatment together, lived in a sober house together, or simply made one another's acquaintance. Other groups are formal and ongoing, such as Alcoholics Anonymous. These groups are critical in replacing the elements of the former social network that facilitated substance use (LaBarre 1964).

Role of Culture in Addiction Prevention

In a multiethnic society like ours, no one preventive strategy is likely to fit all groups. On one hand, some groups might prefer to socialize their members into lifelong abstinence from alcohol. American Indian, Seventh-Day Adventist, and Muslim communities would be examples for this strategy. As noted above, the risk comes if the person from this group joins the mainstream culture, in which alcohol, caffeine, and tobacco are licit substances (Fleming 1992).

Another strategy lies in socializing children and adolescents into healthful patterns of substance usage. The risk is that some percentage of people so socialized will develop substance abuse or dependence as a result of this exposure. Even youthful dependence on caffeine can occur. It may be doubtful whether a healthy use of tobacco—for example via cigarettes—is even feasible for most people given its highly addictive properties.

Locus of Clinical Care

Inpatient

Inpatient care involves considerable medical traditions, so ethnic sensitivity may be difficult to implement. Nonetheless, people who are miserable with opiate or sedative withdrawal may need, and often readily accept, inpatient care. The crucial step occurs in discharge planning, which should begin even before admission to the inpatient setting. Work with the family or community should begin at this phase of treatment. Often a visit from an ethnic or cultural peer from a recovery group or program can be the first step toward recovery.

Consultation-Liaison

The consultant focusing on substance abuse problems may not be welcome to the patient who is being treated on a medical or surgical ward for a substance-related illness. Before the consultation, the attending physician and nurses should tell the patient of their concern about the patient's use of substances and that they are initiating a substance abuse consultation to aid in the patient's assessment and treatment recommendations. Attending clinicians do not always perform this simple courtesy, with the result that the patient is enraged and the consultant becomes a target for hostility. On the other hand, the consultant may be more familiar with substance abuse subcultural issues, which may lead the patient to feel more understood than he or she is by the referring physician.

Outpatient

Increasingly, outpatient consultations and evaluations are becoming the norm. These may take place after an outpatient detoxification or brief care in a detoxification setting. Whenever possible, a family member or close friend who is committed to the patient's recovery should accompany the patient to the visit and should participate as a collateral resource. Especially if the patient and clinician differ in ethnic backgrounds, the presence of an ethnic peer can help in reassuring the patient of an accurate evaluation. If the patient cannot speak English well, a translator from the patient's ethnic background can likewise reassure the patient (Marcos 1979).

Child-Adolescent

Children or young adolescents with a substance abuse problem are highly likely to come from a family in which the single parent, or both parents when present, abuse substances. The child may sneak the parent's substance, such as alcohol, cannabis, or prescription drugs (Swanson et al. 1971). Alternatively, the child may use solvents because these are easily obtained. In addition, there may be a tradition of solvent abuse among youths in the community, as has occurred in communities torn by widespread substance abuse (Kaufman 1973). Acquired mental retardation secondary to solvent abuse should be considered, because special educational and rehabilitation resources may be necessary (Beauvais et al. 1985; Padilla et al. 1979). Children may also be abused or neglected by substance-abusing caregivers—a notable problem in groups with high rates of substance abuse (DeBruyn et al. 1992). Conversely, such groups can become exemplars of healthy child raising with the help of community projects (Kleinfeld 1982).

Geriatric

The role of the elderly person in the ethnic group should be considered. As indicated earlier (see "Case 3: Forty Years of Heavy Drinking"), the family in some groups may be unable to confront a matriarch or patriarch regarding his or her substance abuse. In other groups, the confrontation may go well, as in the following case:

Case 4: An Elderly Man Drowning His Grief in Drink

Mr. Jackson, a 73-year-old African American man, had experienced the death of his wife 10 months earlier. Although Mr. Jackson had drunk heavily for a time in his 20s, he had been abstinent from alcohol while his wife was alive. After her death, Mr. Jackson had constant misery and severe problems with insomnia. Virtually from the day of her death, he began drinking on a daily basis, with amounts increasing as time went by. His children, who visited often, saw severe deterioration in his nutrition, appearance, health, self-care, and living circumstances. Mr. Jackson was admitted to the hospital after a syncopal episode followed by disorientation; dehydration and abnormal liver enzyme values were the only findings. The family proved critical in resolving the problem in a way that was acceptable to all concerned. Mr. Jackson moved into the home of one of his sons, occupying quarters vacated by his now-adult grandchildren. The family involved him in the same round of social affiliations that he had experienced when his wife was alive (e.g., church, community organizations, family events). Mr. Jackson joined a self-help group composed of other elderly men. For several months his psychiatrist assisted him in doing the grief work that substance use had undermined following his wife's death. Mr. Jackson's recovery was steady and uneventful.

Forensic

Forensic cases can test the law as well as clinical and social science. Families and friends may find it acceptable for a Somali immigrant to traffic in khat or a Hmong immigrant to traffic in opium. However, traffickers can expect sanctions from the majority society regardless of ethnic origin or affiliation. Generally, the Immigration and Naturalization Service anticipates such problems and orients immigrants to the laws of their new country. In court cases, the trafficking immigrant cannot successfully plead ignorance or special cultural status. The courts often incarcerate the offender and then deport him or her to the country of origin. If deportation cannot be accomplished and the federal government is involved, the person may be held in detention indefinitely.

Conclusion

Addicts experience a decline in activities reinforcing ethnic identity and supporting ethnic organizations. Recovery involves a cultural component along with physical and psychological components. Elements of cultural recovery involve a viable regained ethnic identity; a functional social network committed to the person's recovery; religious, spiritual, or moral recommitment; recreational or avocational activities; and recovery of social role and status either in the recovering community or in the society at large (or in both).

Especially early in recovery, substitute networks can facilitate full recovery. A subculture of therapists and self-help groups can guide the individual toward health and stability. These recovery subcultures can support, confront, and guide the person in avoiding dangerous situations that might precipitate a relapse.

The recovering person reaches a point where further progress means branching out from the recovery subculture. This movement involves risks: exposure to substance use and potential failure at a new enterprise. If the recovery subculture, composed of both professionals and lay peers, has done its work well, the recovering person should be prepared for this step—often one of the final steps in recovery following years of adjustment to sobriety.

References

Beauvais F, Oetting ER, Edward RW: Trends in the use of inhalants among American Indian adolescents. White Cloud Journal of American Indian Mental Health 3:3–11, 1985

Bergman RL: Navaho peyote use: its apparent safety. Am J Psychiatry 128:695–699, 1971

Brady M: Giving away the grog: an ethnography of Aboriginal drinkers who quit without help. Drug Alcohol Rev 12:401–411, 1993

Caetano R: Acculturation and drinking patterns among U.S. Hispanics. Br J Addict 82:789–799, 1987

Davidson R: Assessment of the alcohol dependence syndrome: a review of self-report screening questionnaires. Br J Clin Psychol 26:243–255, 1987

DeBruyn LM, Lujan CC, May PA: A comparative study of abused and neglected American Indian children in the southwest. Soc Sci Med 35:305–315, 1992

Dumont M: Tavern culture: the sustenance of homeless men. Am J Orthopsychiatry 37:938–945, 1967

Fields A, Tararin PA: Opium in China. Br J Addict 64:371–382, 1970

Fleming CM: The next twenty years of prevention in Indian country: visionary, complex, and practical. Am Indian Alask Native Ment Health Res 4:85–88, 1992

Godlaski TM, Leukefeld C, Cloud R: Recovery: with and without self-help. Subst Use Misuse 32:621–627, 1997

Graves T: Acculturation, access, and alcohol in a tri-ethnic community. Am Anthropol 69:306–321, 1967

Griffiths P, Gossop M, Wickenden S, et al: A transcultural pattern of drug use: qat (khat) in the U.K. Br J Psychiatry 170:281–284, 1997

Hamer JH: Acculturation stress and the functions of alcohol among the Forest Potawatomi. Q J Stud Alcohol 26:285–302, 1965

Husted J, Johnson T, Redwing L: Multi-dimensional adolescent treatment with American Indians. Am Indian Alask Native Ment Health Res 6:23–30, 1995

Jessor R, Graves TD, Hanson RC, et al (eds): Society, Personality and Deviant Behavior: A Study of a Tri-Ethnic Community. New York, Holt, Rinehart, & Winston, 1968

Kaufman A: Gasoline sniffing among children in a Pueblo Indian village. Pediatrics 51:1060–1065, 1973

Kennedy JG, Teague J, Fairbanks L: Qat use in North Yemen and the problem of addiction: a study in medical anthropology. Cult Med Psychiatry 4:311–344, 1980

Kleinfeld J: Getting it together at adolescence: case studies of positive socializing environments for Eskimo youth, in New Directions in Prevention Among American Indian and Alaska Native Communities. Edited by Manson SM. Portland, OR, University of Oregon, 1982, pp 341–365

Kraus RF, Buffler PA: Sociocultural stress and the American Native in Alaska: an analysis of changing patterns of psychiatric illness and alcohol abuse among Alaska Natives. Cult Med Psychiatry 3:111–151, 1979

LaBarre W: The Peyote Cult. Hamden, CT, Shoe String Press, 1964

Marcos LR: Effects of interpreters on the evaluation of psychopathology in non-English-speaking patients. Am J Psychiatry 136:171–174, 1979

Markides KS: Acculturation and alcohol consumption among Mexican Americans: a three-generation study. Am J Public Health 78:1178–1181, 1988

Martin J, Zweben JE: Addressing treatment needs of Southeast Asian Mien opium users in California. J Psychoactive Drugs 25:73–76, 1993

Mayfield D, McLeod G, Hall P: The CAGE questionnaire: validation of a new alcoholism screening instrument. Am J Psychiatry 131:1121–1123, 1974

Murphy JM: Psychiatric labeling in cross-cultural perspective. Science 191:1019–1028, 1976

Padilla ER, Padilla AM, Morales A, et al: Inhalant, marijuana and alcohol abuse among barrio children and adolescents. Int J Addict 14:945–964, 1979

Red Horse Y: A cultural network model: perspectives for adolescent services and para-professional training, in New Directions in Prevention Among American Indian and Alaska Native Communities. Edited by Manson S. Portland, OR, University of Oregon, 1982, pp 173–185

Robin RW, Long JC, Rasmussen JK, et al: Relationship of binge drinking to alcohol dependence, other psychiatric disorders, and behavioral problems in an American Indian tribe. Alcohol Clin Exp Res 22:518–523, 1998

Rodin AE: Infants and gin mania in 18th century London. JAMA 245:1237–1239, 1981

Selzer M: The Michigan Alcoholism Screening Test (MAST): the quest for a new diagnostic instrument. Am J Psychiatry 127:1653–1658, 1971

Stull DD: Victims of modernization: accident rates and Papago Indian adjustment. Hum Organ 31:227–240, 1972

Sutker PB, Archer RP, Allain AN: Psychopathology of drug abusers: sex and ethnic considerations. Int J Addict 15:605–613, 1980

Swanson DW, Bratrude AP, Brown EM: Alcohol abuse in a population of Indian children. Dis Nerv Syst 32:835–842, 1971

Taylor V: The triumph of the Alkali Lake Indian band. Alcohol Health Res World 11(3):57, 1987

Weibel-Orlando JC: Pass the bottle, bro!: a comparison of urban and rural Indian drinking patterns, in Alcohol Use Among U.S. Ethnic Minorities. Edited by Spiegler DL, Tate D, Aitken S, et al. Washington, DC, U.S. Department of Health and Human Services, 1985, pp 269–287

Westermeyer J: Opium dens: a social resource for addicts in Laos. Arch Gen Psychiatry 31:237–240, 1974

Westermeyer J: Ethnic factors in psychopathology and substance abuse, in Substance Abuse and Psychopathology. Edited by Alterman AI. New York, Plenum, 1983, pp 45–68

Westermeyer J: Psychiatric diagnosis across cultural boundaries. Am J Psychiatry 142:798–805, 1985

Westermeyer J: Cultural factors in clinical assessment. J Consult Clin Psychol 55:471–478, 1987

Westermeyer J: Mental Health for Refugees and Other Migrants: Social and Preventative Approaches. Springfield, IL, Charles C Thomas, 1989a

Westermeyer J: Monitoring recovery from substance abuse: rationales, methods and challenges. Adv Alcohol Subst Abuse 8:93–106, 1989b

Westermeyer J: Historical-social context of psychoactive substance disorders, in Clinical Textbook of Addiction Disorders. Edited by Francis R, Miller S. New York, Guilford, 1992, pp 23–40

Westermeyer J: The role of cultural and social factors in the cause of addictive disorders. Psychiatr Clin North Am 22:253–273, 1999

Westermeyer J, Neider J: Social network and psychopathology among substance abusers. Am J Psychiatry 145:1265–1269, 1988

Westermeyer J, Walker D: Approaches to treatment of alcoholism across cultural boundaries. Psychiatr Ann 12:434–439, 1982

Westermeyer J, Lyfoung T, Westermeyer M, et al: Opium addiction among Indochinese refugees in the United States: characteristics of addicts and their opium use. Am J Drug Alcohol Abuse 17:267–277, 1991

Zimberg S: Evaluation of alcoholism treatment in Harlem. Q J Stud Alcohol 35:550–557, 1974

7

Culture and Forensic Psychiatry

Daryl Matthews, M.D., Ph.D.
Wen-Shing Tseng, M.D.

Forensic psychiatry is a unique subspecialty of psychiatry at the interface of psychiatry and the law. Its function is to provide psychiatric expertise for a society's dispute-resolution and criminal justice systems. To carry out this function properly and relevantly in a multicultural society, the practice of forensic psychiatry should be culturally informed.

Forensic psychiatry is oriented to careful psychiatric evaluation, and in contemporary American psychiatry a careful evaluation includes attention to sociocultural factors. In its *Practice Guideline for Psychiatric Evaluation of Adults*, the American Psychiatric Association (1995) recommends the inclusion of sociocultural issues in the evaluation process, including the assessment of issues pertaining to "culture, ethnicity, gender, sexual orientation…religious/spiritual beliefs, social class, and physical and social environment influencing the patient's symptoms and behavior" (p. 16).

As forensic psychiatry develops, it is likely that sociocultural concerns will take greater prominence in the discipline. This is because of the development of increased academic interest in cultural forensic psychiatry, demographic changes occurring in the United States, and increasing professional attention being given to diversity in American society across disciplines.

Culture, Law, and the Legal System

In some societies, torture and execution are routinely practiced within the bounds of the legal system (Amnesty International 2002). Major areas of civil litigation in the United States are unknown in other countries. There are enormous international and cross-cultural variations of every aspect of law and the legal system: what constitutes a crime, standards for arrest, rights of detainees, role of the judge, availability of trial by jury, and every aspect of legal procedure across civil, criminal, and family law. The legal system of a country, the expression of political and historical forces, is also profoundly shaped by social and cultural factors (Chaleby 1996). Ciccone and Ferracuti (1995) have called for an expanded understanding of comparative cross-national forensic psychiatry.

In this chapter we consider forensic psychiatry only in the context of the system of laws in the United States; however, it is essential to understand that evaluees' responses to the U.S. legal system may be based in part on expectations shaped by the legal system of their nation or culture of origin. In the most extreme manifestation of this, individuals who have grown up under or have experienced the consequences of a repressive legal system may assume that the U.S. legal system and its personnel, including the forensic evaluator, operate in the same manner. Questions by the examiner may be interpreted as hostile and interrogative, and the examiner himself or herself may be seen as sadistic or voyeuristic. There may be high levels of mistrust of physicians involved in the legal system (Physicians for Human Rights 2001). Forensic psychiatrists themselves may be viewed with suspicion due to psychiatric abuses in the examinee's country of origin (Human Rights Watch and Geneva Initiative on Psychiatry 2002). These responses must be interpreted in the context of the culture of origin of the evaluee; otherwise one is at risk of inappropriately concluding that the evaluee is unduly guarded, suspicious, paranoid, or even delusional.

This concern applies even to cultural variations within the United States. Our educational system fosters an idealized and unrealistic view of the U.S. criminal justice system, which may be further reinforced by inaccurate media portrayals. For example, the extent to which our system produces and tolerates wide disparities in access to competent counsel and expert witnesses, the extent to which penal outcomes are highly correlated with race and social class, and the crucial role of the plea bargain in our justice system are not widely appreciated in American society. However, these points may be very salient to members of the social groups most commonly injured by such practices: the poor and members of racial and ethnic minorities.

Is it paranoid or is it accurate for an indigent defendant to assert: "I don't trust my lawyer; he's overworked, has no personal interest in my case, works for the government, is a friend of the prosecutor, and did not meet with me personally until my arraignment." Is this a sign of a cynical but correct understanding of the U.S. legal system, consistent with the defendant's sociocultural background, or is it undue suspiciousness? The answer is important, because a "rational ability to assist defense counsel" is a constitutional requirement for trial competency in all U.S. jurisdictions (*Dusky v. United States*). Without more evidence of mental disorder, the correct answer is probably that this view is cultural rather than psychopathological; however, novice examiners frequently overlook the former in favor of the latter.

Even supposedly objective psychological test instruments in the forensic context may incorporate these cultural biases. For example, the Competency Screening Test has been criticized for being biased against defendants with a negative view of the legal system. Individuals who express cynicism about the criminal justice process could be incorrectly scored as incompetent, contributing to the test's undesirably high false-positive rate (Melton et al. 1997).

Forensic psychiatry is concerned with a wide variety of psycholegal issues and types of evaluations, ranging from assessments of mental state at the time of an alleged criminal offense to determinations of the capacity to make a will or to function as a parent. In each setting in which forensic psychiatric expertise is called for, consideration of sociocultural factors should be part of the assessment process (Tseng et al. 2004).

In the sections that follow we present (without attempting to be systematic or exhaustive) examples of the interrelationship between culture and psycholegal decision making.

Forensic Issues and Culture

Is There a Mental Disorder?

In any psychiatric assessment, clinical judgments of normality or pathology require a cultural perspective. This is particularly crucial in forensic psychiatry, however, because the consequences of such judgments may be so profound. On the basis of forensic assessments, individuals may win or lose significant disability benefits, retain or lose custody of their children, be sent to prison rather than hospitalized, and, in the most extreme cases, be found competent to receive the death penalty. Furthermore, in many clinical situations the psychiatrist will have the opportunity to observe the patient longitudinally; forensic assessments instead often involve a single opportunity to interview the evaluee. This compounds the need to routinely consider cultural issues in every forensic evaluation.

The professional culture of psychology and psychiatry has permeated American society. Popular American explanations for behavior at the time of this writing include attention-deficit/hyperactivity disorder; dissociative identity disorder; medication side effects; and various addictions to drugs, sex, and gambling. Yet there is continued and vigorous debate in the mental health disciplines about how to regard such conditions from the perspective of legal responsibility and other issues intrinsic to the resolution of legal disputes (Bonnie 2002; Piper 1996; Saks and Behnke 1997). Therefore, the evaluator must not take at face value attributions of illness or causation offered by the various participants in the legal process. This applies not only to minority cultures but also to the dominant culture in the United States. The forensic evaluator must look well beyond culturally stereotyped notions of the causes of behavior, including stereotypes that may have been perpetuated by the professions themselves (Horwitz 2002).

Culturally sound forensic assessments are especially difficult for certain kinds of psychopathology, such as delusions (Levy 1996). For a belief to qualify as delusional according to DSM-IV-TR, it must be one that is "not…ordinarily accepted by other members of the person's culture or subculture" (American Psychiatric Association 2000, p. 821). Therefore, in assessing the psychopathology of an evaluee's belief, the evaluator must know enough about the evaluee's culture and the extent of the evaluee's participation in it to make this determination. In gathering such evidence, of special importance is obtaining relevant cultural information from family members, friends, or other individuals in the community of the same ethnic or cultural background as the evaluee. Consultation with a clinician who is familiar with the language and culture of the evaluee may be helpful in some instances as well. Similar concerns may apply in evaluating the presence or absence of other psychopathological features such as hallucinations, flashbacks, or dissociation.

Included in Appendix I of DSM-IV-TR is the "Outline for Cultural Formulation," a useful tool for systematically thinking through the variety of modes whereby cultural factors may affect the psychiatric status of an individual. In litigation in which cultural influences may be prominent, use of this guide helps assure the evaluator and can demonstrate to the judge and jury that the full range of possibilities pertaining to culture and the present evaluation issue have been considered.

Culture-Related Specific Syndromes and Criminal Behavior

Culture-related specific syndromes (Tseng 2001), also called culture-bound syndromes, are psychiatric disorders that are closely related to a particular culture and that manifest a unique clinical picture not described in regular classifications of psychiatric disorders. These syndromes are sometimes associated with criminal behavior. Descriptions include episodic, sudden homicidal behavior (such as in amok) (Hatta 1996; Hempel et al. 2000), criminal behavior occurring during a dissociated or possessed state (such as malignant latah) (Woon 1988; Zhang 1992), or culturally associated murder/suicide behavior by a family (such as ikashinjiu in Japan, which is parental double suicide associated with child homicide) (Ohara 1963; Tseng and Matthews, in press).

A thorough forensic evaluation of an individual with an apparent mental disorder may require consideration of the possibility that he or she is experiencing a culture-related specific syndrome. Reflecting a view propounded by Tseng (2001a), Kleinman (1980), and others, Schultz-Ross (1997) suggested that "symptoms are to be interpreted within a cultural context, and cultural cause excluded before the label of psychopathology is given" (p. 181). Because many culture-specific syndromes involve forensically relevant issues such as violence, dissociation, and attributions of nonresponsibility, this dictum applies with special force in forensic cases.

Evaluation of Criminal Responsibility

Although an individual's views of responsibility will generally not affect a court's determination of responsibility, they may affect such forensically important issues as feelings and expressions of remorse, courtroom behavior and demeanor, and judicial determinations of culpability.

For example, the extent to which an examinee views responsibility for one's conduct as an individual or collective matter deserves careful consideration from a cultural perspective. The deviant individual is the sole person on whom responsibility devolves in an individually oriented society, so when an adult commits an offense, his parents, spouse, or children do not share the responsibility for the wrongful behavior. However, in a family- or group-oriented society, responsibility does not necessarily end with the individual. A person's legal or financial debt may need to be discharged by his parents, spouse, or children. For example, in India, a highly family-oriented society, legal responsibility for a sexual assault may be borne by the perpetrator's family as well as the offender himself, and the shame resulting from the crime may be borne by the victim's family as well as the victim herself (Roth and Pruett 2000).

Case 1: Let the Seller Beware

A 24-year-old Pacific Island man, Mr. Lautusi, was charged with driving without a state auto safety inspection sticker. On questioning by the judge, Mr. Lautusi revealed that he had very recently purchased the car from a man who had lied to him about its condition. The seller had represented that the car would be able to pass the safety inspection, but this was not so. Mr. Lautusi believed this to be a reasonable defense to the charge; his assertion was that the seller was responsible for the car's not passing inspection. The judge spent some time explaining the Western concept of *caveat emptor* to Mr. Lautusi. She also stated that she was showing leniency toward the defendant based on his cultural perspective, and significantly reduced the fine levied for the offense. Mr. Lautusi, however, remained firm in his assertion that the court was treating him unjustly.

A frequent task in forensic psychiatry is to provide consultation to the legal system regarding whether a mentally ill defendant was able at the time of an alleged offense to know or appreciate that his behavior was wrong. However, it is important for the evaluator to recognize that conceptions of "right" and "wrong" are not only defined by the legal system but also shaped by culture. The meaning of these concepts is not absolute and may vary from society to society. Individuals' assessments of wrongfulness will depend on cultural views of the intention and meaning of the action taken, implications of its consequences, and how others perceive the behavior in society. For instance, stealing a loaf of bread for a starving nephew may be considered very wrong and deserving of substantial punishment (as described in Victor Hugo's *Les Miserables*) or may be regarded as a minor infraction necessitating only a small sanction. Individuals learn to judge wrongfulness as part of their acculturation, and the developed standards of wrongfulness vary across societies and cultures. This fact is of particular importance in jurisdictions where case law provides—to forensic evaluator and jury alike—no guidance on the meaning of wrongfulness.

Lying, Manipulation, and Malingering

To defend one's behavior, secure benefit, avoid punishment, or seek better treatment, one may deny, distort, or rationalize the situation relating to the occurrence of criminal actions, one's mental or physical condition, or similar matters. This occurrence may be detected and interpreted by others as lying, manipulating, or malingering, depending on the nature of the behavior. In some cultures, such behavior may be condemned, and the individual engaging in it may be regarded as not credible on other issues. In other cultures, such behavior is understood and tolerated as more or less acceptable and is not viewed so harshly.

Individuals who come from a society where authority is harsh and punishment cruel (for example, persons who grew up in the former Soviet Union) may have learned from childhood, as a survival skill, to use distortion or deception as a means of dealing with an intolerable political or social situation. Important streams in American society, in contrast, may hold that to be "honest" even in the face of punishment is a virtue, as exemplified by the childhood story of George Washington and the cherry tree; to be *dis*honest is considered unreliable and disgraceful. Individuals' attitudes toward truth and deception are of significance in the psychiatric assessment of malingering. These attitudes in turn must be understood and evaluated from the perspective of the cultural norm that underlies them. This cultural aspect contributes to the difficulty in assessing evaluees for malingering and deception (Bunnting et al. 1996).

Involuntary Hospitalization, Institutionalization, and Discharge

The frequency of involuntary admissions to psychiatric hospitals varies considerably among countries (Riecher-Rössler and Rössler 1993). It is most closely related to varying legal standards for commitment across different societies. However, rates of involuntary hospitalization also vary among individuals of different ethnic backgrounds living in the same society (Thomas et al. 1993). These rates may vary in part because clinicians' ascriptions of dangerousness may be biased in assessing members of ethnic groups other than their own. Also, depending on an individual's cultural background, threatening behavior may be more or less associated with actual violence. Therefore, the need for involuntary admission requires careful evaluation from a cultural perspective in addition to psychological, medical, legal, and ethical considerations.

Whether a person can be safely discharged from a hospital or released from prison may demand a careful cultural evaluation. In addition to assessment of the individual's psychiatric condition, assessment of social safety and the reaction of others in the community to the potential release is needed before a release decision can be made. Whether the individual can be accepted by his or her family and reintegrated into the community—whether the person can secure a job, develop appropriate interpersonal relations, be supported in receiving treatment, refrain from substance abuse, and learn how to detect signs of relapse— may, in individual cases, depend in good measure on social and cultural factors. These include reactions by family and community members to illness and deviant behavior.

Conducting a Culturally Competent Forensic Psychiatric Evaluation

Evaluation Methods

Because their purpose is different from that of clinical evaluations, forensic evaluations require a different method than clinical assessments (Melton et al. 1997). If the evaluation involves an examinee who is from a different ethnic or cultural background than the examiner, many of the issues pertinent to transcultural clinical assessments would apply (Tseng 2001). The establishment of a proper relationship with the defendant, the maintenance of rapport within the confines of neutrality, and the encouragement of the examinee to provide accurate background information are aspects of a competent forensic evaluation. These issues are all subject to cultural influences.

A special effort is needed for defendants who are unfamiliar with the U.S. legal system. Without an appropriate cultural assessment, for example, individuals who are merely uninformed about their legal rights, legal procedures, and court personnel can be erroneously assessed as incompetent to stand trial. True incompetence requires lack of ability to learn about these matters rather than simply lack of current understanding (Grisso 1988).

These concerns also apply to psychological testing. Determining whether or not the test instruments are cross-culturally reliable and valid may require careful review of the relevant psychometric literature. How the defendant understands the purposes, procedures, and meaning of psychological tests and how he or she reacts to their administration also deserve careful consideration. Some examinees, due to lack of familiarity with psychological testing or misunderstanding of the meaning or use of such measurements, may perform in such a way that the results are distorted or invalid. These situations require special efforts to provide explanation and guidance to the evaluee. Finally, particular attention is needed when interpreting the data obtained and developing conclusions (Tseng 2001).

Translators

Forensic psychiatric assessment relies on interviews of the evaluee as a major source of information, and the needed information is acquired through the process of communication in the interview. Therefore, the lack of a shared language between evaluator and evaluee poses a significant challenge in carrying out the forensic interview. Even though a translator can be utilized, communication is still subject to limitations and the possibilities of distortion and misunderstanding. Although this is true for clinical assessments as well as forensic assessments, the impact of the latter on the individual may be more profound, because the results of the examination may determine the outcome of the legal decision: the death penalty or psychiatric hospitalization, a sentence of 3 years or 30 years in prison, or loss of custody of a child. Extra effort is therefore necessary to avoid a mistake that will produce an incorrect outcome.

It is well known that different languages use different sets of vocabulary to express meaning. One language may have a limited vocabulary to describe a concept, whereas another language might have many differentiated words to elaborate on it. For example, Micronesian people have many words for *cloud*, depending on the type of cloud, whereas English has only the one noun. The same situation occurs in language related to behavior or emotion. For the indulgent love between child and parent, Japanese people use several different words centering around the key word *amae*—which literally means "sweet"—to elaborate the delicate, permitted affection between parent and child. This basic, benevolent, dependent affection is highly valued in Japanese culture (Doi 1962). In Western languages, there is difficulty finding an equivalent word to *amae*, and there is difficulty in properly translating that Japanese word into English.

The impact of this phenomenon on forensic practice may be great. For instance, words used by a non-English-speaking defendant in his or her native language to mean "I hit him on the head and he died" might be interpreted simply as "I killed him" by an unskillful or inexperienced translator. Such a translation could have a significantly different implication from a legal perspective. Even for an experienced and skillful translator, it often becomes a challenge to interpret a word from one language to another not only as accurately as possible, but also in a culturally equivalent manner. Issues of provocation, self-defense, justification, motivation, and causation due to mental illness may potentially be obscured by incorrect translations of the defendant's description of his own behavior.

Proper selection of the translator, in addition to adequate orientation and guidance by the evaluator, is desirable. The translator must not only be competent in language, but ideally should have knowledge relating to psychiatry, culture and behavior, and the legal system. This also applies to individuals who prepare written translations of documents. Evaluators should also be alert to issues of countertransference in interpreters who work in the legal system; these issues can result in subtle deviations from a neutral interpreting role (Mellman 1995). The outcome may otherwise be erroneous. The following case example provides an illustration of the problems of language in cross-cultural assessment in forensic psychiatry.

Case 2: The Power of Words Lost in Translation

In sworn court testimony, a Chinese male defendant, Mr. Li Ming, complained about how he had been mistreated by his boss. He described his boss as always shouting at him and swearing "[I will] fuck your mother's vagina!" The Chinese-speaking interpreter, being reluctant to make a literal translation of what Mr. Ming said, simply translated that the boss spoke "dirty words" to the defendant. The interpreter, a highly educated, well-mannered woman, refused to repeat the actual, quite disgraceful expression in front of others in court. As a result, the translation did not depict the actual expression complained about by the defendant, as an explanation for his subsequent violent behavior against his boss; it failed to communicate the full weight and gravity of the insult. Thus, Mr. Ming was less able to effectively explain his behavior to the court and in turn was significantly less able to influence its decision making.

Evaluees' Interpretations of Motivation and Behavior

Part of one's culture is the rules and guidelines one follows in manifesting behavior. Behavior that is prohibited in one culture may be viewed as permissible or even desirable and encouraged in another. For example, in matrilineal Micronesian culture (tracing descent through the maternal line rather than the paternal, as in a patrilineal system), the brother-sister relationship is considered the most important bond in family relations. As a result, there is a strong taboo against close physical contact between a brother and sister. Traditionally, the taboo is observed to such an extent that a brother and sister are not allowed in the same room together when there is no other person present; one of them must leave the room immediately. From a psychological and functional perspective, this taboo exists to protect the close relationship between them. In other cultures the concept of premarital virginity is not emphasized. Young people are permitted to have sexual relations, and even to bear children, before a formal marriage. Within such cultural systems, what is a "normal" or "unusual" relationship between men and women needs careful interpretation.

The entire pattern of communication, interaction, and relationships between men and women is influenced by cultural factors, which may require careful assessment and understanding in a legal situation. For example, when a person says "I like you" to a person of the opposite sex, or shakes hands or hugs a person of the opposite sex as a social greeting, or telephones someone of the opposite sex at night (irrespective of the purpose of the call), the meaning to the individuals involved requires careful scrutiny. When a woman complains that she was "seduced," "sexually harassed," or "sexually assaulted," her meaning deserves careful analysis and understanding before any interpretations or judgments are made. One's interpretation should draw from the cultural perspective of both the alleged victim and the alleged perpetrator. This is particularly true if the complainant and the accused are of different ethnic, racial, or cultural backgrounds, in which case the situation needs consideration from the perspectives of both cultures for the intercultural interaction that took place to be understood. The following case involves intercultural issues in relationships between the sexes.

Case 3: Cultural Misunderstanding or Erotic Delusion?

A psychiatrist was asked by a hospital to evaluate a female Asian nurse, Miss Mei-mei, who believed that a Caucasian male doctor working in the same hospital was in love with her. She persisted in contacting the doctor and behaved in such a way that he complained to the hospital administrator. Assessment revealed that the nurse had emigrated from a conservative and traditional Asian country to the United States a year earlier. Her command of English was barely sufficient for her work as a nurse, and she lacked social experience in the host society. In the interview, she asserted that the doctor had clearly indicated his affection to her, leading her to eventually believe that he was in love with her. She related that the doctor, who lived in the hospital dormitory next door to her, always gave her a big smile and asked "How are you today" when they encountered each other in the building. She explained that, in her home country, a man never asks such a "personal" question about a woman unless he is romantically interested in her. Beyond that, on one occasion he knocked on her door to borrow sugar for his coffee. She explained that, in her country, a man does not make such an excuse to "intrude" into a woman's private life unless he has romantic intentions. She listed other "evidence" that he had displayed his romantic attraction to her. For example, he had asked for her apartment phone number, and called her one time for some trivial matter. After she came to believe that he was in love with her, she became upset one day when she found out he was dating another woman. She then felt that she had been betrayed by him and, in her anger, she called him to annoy him.

It was the psychiatrist's challenge to find out whether this was merely an intercultural misunderstanding related to the expression of affection between the man and woman, or if it was associated with an erotomanic delusion or other psychopathological features on the part of the nurse. Clinical information, her history, her personality and behavior pattern in general, and her relationships with others (particularly with men in working and social situations) were all helpful in comprehensively assessing the case. But also of major assistance was consultation with other women from the same cultural background as the nurse.

Examiners' Interpretations of Motivation and Behavior

Just as the evaluee may misinterpret behavior based on cultural differences, so may the psychiatrist, attorney, judge, or jury. All will react to the psychiatric findings not based solely on technical and professional information, but also from the perspective of their cultural background, which may be quite different from that of the evaluee.

In the case example below, a woman alleged that she had been raped by her boss but did not reveal the incident to anyone—including her own husband—at the time, and instead first made a complaint almost a year later. How should her "delaying" the accusation be interpreted by attorneys, judge, or jury? This depends on the woman's cultural background.

Case 4: Why the Delay?

A middle-aged married woman, Mrs. Mariko Smith, alleged in a civil action that her boss had raped her almost a year earlier. She made no complaint at the time of the incident and did not even inform her husband. She told her attorney that in the month before her allegation a female co-worker revealed to her that she also been raped by the boss. The woman said she became very angry and decided, along with her co-worker, to take legal action against their boss. Her attorney, concerned about why she had delayed making the accusation, sought psychiatric consultation.

History from Mrs. Smith revealed that she came to the United States from Japan two decades earlier. She married a local man who was more than 15 years older than she. She had no children, but she said her husband was kind to her and that they have had a good marital relationship. Her husband was already retired and was financially dependent on her income from work.

Her English was just sufficient for her work in the small retail shop in which she was employed. Her boss was a married man, originally from Asia himself. He had two or three women employees, all Asian immigrants.

Mrs. Smith said that about 1 year previously, her boss asked her to work late one evening, as he often did. When she was alone with him, he asked her to come into his office and sat next to her on the sofa. He began caressing her and eventually removed her clothes and initiated sexual intercourse. She was surprised about what was happening but was too frightened to resist, run, or shout for help, since, according to her, he was physically very strong and there was no way to resist or escape. Besides, she added, he was, after all, her boss. She explained that where she was raised it was not proper for a woman to say no to a man in authority.

After this incident occurred, she did not dare mention it to her husband, for fear that he might divorce her. In her home country, she said, a husband has the right to desert his wife when she has been "contaminated" by another man. Besides, she needed the job to support her family, and there was no easy way for her to find another job. She therefore kept silent about the incident and continued to work at the shop, although making an effort to avoid any opportunity for her boss to take advantage of her again.

Things continued uneventfully until, a month before her complaint, she noticed a recently hired female co-worker—who was much younger and was also an immigrant from Asia—crying at work. Upon her inquiry, the co-worker revealed to her that the boss had raped her as well, in almost the same manner. She became very angry about the fact that her boss had taken advantage of another innocent young woman. Without hesitation this time, she decided to take legal action to punish this behavior.

Seeking Cultural Consultation

When examiner and examinee are from significantly different cultural backgrounds, a cultural consultation may assist in minimizing misunderstandings and misinterpretations of evidence. It is desirable that the forensic evaluator have some familiarity with the cultural background of the client. For this reason, to have an evaluator of the same racial or ethnic background as the evaluee can be advantageous in the practice of forensic psychiatry (Griffith 1998). However, cultural psychiatrists also pointed out that matching the ethnic, racial, or cultural background alone is not usually possible, is not necessarily sufficient, and is not the only solution. Lu (2003), for example, noted that he, as a United States–born psychiatrist of Chinese descent, would have some difficulty understanding the cultural background of a newly arrived immigrant from China. Also, there may be disadvantages to an evaluation conducted by a member of the same ethnic or racial background as the evaluee, particularly someone from the same community (see Chapter 1, Introduction: Culture and Psychiatry). In the forensic context, there is the potential for the evaluator to overidentify with the evaluee, posing a threat to the objectivity of the assessment.

From a practical perspective, it may be helpful to seek assistance in carrying out a forensic evaluation, either as a consultation or as a collaboration, from a psychiatrist or other mental health clinician who is familiar with the examinee's cultural background—particularly when the ethnic, racial, or cultural background of the defendant is a significant issue in the litigation. This may enhance the accuracy of the result. It may influence the direction and course of the investigation, the interpretation of the information obtained, the ultimate diagnosis, and the medicolegal conclusions.

Case 5: A Useful Cultural Consultation

A 38-year-old Filipino woman, Mrs. Cabuang, who was employed as a hospital housekeeper, developed severe depression, multiple somatic symptoms, and spells of moaning and wailing after being questioned by her supervisor about some items that had been stolen from a patient's room. The supervisor had also asked to search Mrs. Cabuang's purse. Her fellow housekeepers who were on duty at the time were also questioned and searched. Although the investigation was reported by all as being cordial and good-natured, Mrs. Cabuang subsequently developed the depressive symptoms. She filed a worker's compensation claim, and an independent medical examination was conducted. The examiner's initial impression was of malingering. However, consultation with a Filipino psychiatrist revealed that in this woman's culture the supervisor's suspicion was something that brought great shame and disgrace on her. The examiner was able to revise his opinions to reflect these cultural issues.

Suggestions for Clinical Practice

1. *Be aware of the increasing expectation of cultural competence.* Psychiatrists who conduct forensic evaluations should routinely consider the contribution of cultural influences to diagnosis and medicolegal conclusions. Although the prime reason for so doing is to ensure the accuracy of the outcome, evaluators may be putting themselves at medicolegal risk should they fail to do so. Although they are normally not subject to malpractice actions by evaluees, forensic psychiatrists are experiencing increased litigation in recent years. In a review of legal liability issues in forensic evaluations, Binder (2002)

described a case in which a psychiatrist conducted a fitness-for-duty evaluation of an employee. The employer's concern was "that the employee often misconstrued actions or conversations to be about himself when they were not," along with a concern about possible violence. The psychiatrist, who diagnosed paranoid personality disorder, was subsequently sued after the woman hired a psychiatrist who opined that the employee's misconstructions were related to cultural issues rather than to mental disorder. The lawsuit was ultimately dismissed, but only "after several years of aggravation and stress for the psychiatrist/defendant."

These concerns apply in correctional and security (forensic) hospital settings. Weinstein (2002) pointed out that the failure on the part of mental health personnel in these settings to overcome the consequences of cultural differences may even be considered patient mistreatment. Cultural competence in medicine has increasingly become an issue among governmental, educational, and professional organizations; standard-setting bodies are increasingly considering cultural competence as being necessary to the practice of the various medical specialties (Accreditation Council for Graduate Medical Education 2000; Center for Mental Health Services 2001).

2. *Consider the ethical implications of cultural competence.* There may even be an ethical basis for culturally competent forensic practice. Griffith (1998) highlighted the necessity for forensic psychiatric ethics to be culturally grounded: "The forensic psychiatrist must seek the psychological and sociocultural truth about the subject and his behavior. This search must be fueled by a profound respect for the subject as a person."

3. *Know what you do not know.* It is important to recall, as Griffith (1998) stated, that "mastery of the evaluation of certain minority groups does not mean mastery of all minority groups." Asian Americans and Pacific Islanders alone are said to comprise more than 43 separate ethnic subgroups (Lu et al. 2002). A clinician with a strong cultural focus and considerable expertise in the evaluation of Asians and Pacific Islanders does not necessarily have such expertise in the evaluation of each different ethnic subgroup within this group, not to mention the assessment of entirely different ethnic groups, such as African Americans or Hispanic Americans. As Lu (2003) observed, "Cultural humility is the road to cultural competence."

References

Accreditation Council for Graduate Medical Education: Program Requirements for Residency Training in Psychiatry. Chicago, IL, Accreditation Council for Graduate Medical Education, 2000. Available at: http://www.acgme.org/ RRC/Psy_Req.asp. Accessed January 28, 2004.

American Psychiatric Association: Practice Guideline for Psychiatric Evaluation of Adults. Washington, DC, American Psychiatric Association, 1995

American Psychiatric Association: Diagnostic and Statistical Manual of Mental Disorders, 4th Edition, Text Revision. Washington, DC, American Psychiatric Association, 2000

Amnesty International: Report 2002. London, Amnesty International, 2002. Available at: http://web.amnesty.org/web/ar2002.nsf/home/home. Accessed January 28, 2004.

Binder RL: Liability for the psychiatrist expert witness. Am J Psychiatry 159:1819–1825, 2002

Bonnie RJ: Responsibility for addiction. J Am Acad Psychiatry Law 30:405–413, 2002

Bunnting BG, Wessels WH, Lasich AJ, et al: The distinction of malingering and mental illness in black forensic cases. Med Law 15:241–247, 1996

Center for Mental Health Services: Cultural Competence Standards in Managed Care Mental Health Services: Four Underserved/Underrepresented Racial/ Ethnic Groups. Washington, DC, Substance Abuse and Mental Health Services Administration, 2001

Chaleby KS: Issues in forensic psychiatry in Islamic jurisprudence. Bull Am Acad Psychiatry Law 24:117–124, 1996

Ciccone JR, Ferracuti S: Comparative forensic psychiatry, I: commentary on the Italian system. Bull Am Acad Psychiatry Law 23:449–452, 1995

Doi T: *Amae:* a key concept for understanding Japanese personality structure, in Japanese Culture: Its Development and Characteristics. Edited by Smith RJ, Beardsley RK. Chicago, IL, Aldine, 1962, pp 132–139

Dusky v United States, 362 US 402 (1960)

Griffith EE: Ethics in forensic psychiatry: a cultural response to Stone and Appelbaum. J Am Acad Psychiatry Law 26:171–184, 1998

Grisso T: Competency to Stand Trial Evaluation: A Manual for Practice. Sarasota, FL, Professional Resource Exchange, 1988

Hatta SM: A Malay cross-cultural worldview and forensic review of amok. Aust N Z J Psychiatry 30:505–510, 1996

Hempel AG, Levine RE, Meloy JR, et al: A cross-cultural review of sudden mass assault by a single individual in the Oriental and Occidental cultures. J Forensic Sci 45:582–588, 2000

Human Rights Watch and Geneva Initiative on Psychiatry: Dangerous Minds: Political Psychiatry in China Today and Its Origins in the Mao Era. New York, Human Rights Watch, 2002

Horwitz AV: Creating Mental Illness. Chicago, IL, University of Chicago Press, 2002

Kleinman A: Patients and Healers in the Context of Culture: An Exploration of the Borderland Between Anthropology, Medicine, and Psychiatry. Berkeley, CA, University of California Press, 1980

Levy A: Forensic implications of the difficulties of defining delusions. Med Law 15:257–260, 1996

Lu F: Cultural competence: clinical, training and systems perspectives. Oral presentation at Grand Rounds, Department of Psychiatry, John A. Burns School of Medicine, University of Hawaii at Manoa, Honolulu, Hawaii, January 31, 2003

Lu F, Du N, Gaw A, et al: A psychiatric residency curriculum about Asian-American issues. Acad Psychiatry 26:225–236, 2002

Mellman LA: Countertransference in court interpreters. Bull Am Acad Psychiatry Law 23:367–471, 1995

Melton GB, Petrila J, Poythreas NG, et al: Psychological Evaluations for the Courts: A Handbook for Mental Health Professionals and Lawyers, 2nd Edition. New York, Guilford, 1997

Ohara K: Characteristics of suicide in Japan, especially of parent-child double suicide. Am J Psychiatry 120:382–385, 1963

Physicians for Human Rights: Examining Asylum Seekers: A Health Professional's Guide to Medical and Psychological Evaluations of Torture. Boston, MA, Physicians for Human Rights, 2001

Piper A: Hoax and Reality: The Bizarre World of Multiple Personality Disorder. Northvale, NJ, Jason Aronson, 1996

Riecher-Rossler A, Rossler W: Compulsory admission of psychiatric patients: an international comparison. Acta Psychiatr Scand 87:231–236, 1993

Roth JA, Pruett MK: America's daughters on Ghandi's daughters. J Am Acad Psychiatry Law 28:352–356, 2000

Saks ER, Behnke SH: Jekyll on Trial: Multiple Personality Disorder and the Criminal Law. New York, New York University Press, 1997

Schultz-Ross RA: Violent behavior, in Culture and Psychopathology: A Guide to Clinical Assessment. Edited by Tseng WS, Streltzer J. New York, Brunner/Mazel, 1997, pp 173–189

Thomas CS, Stone K, Osborn M, et al: Psychiatric morbidity and compulsory admission among UK-born Europeans, Afro-Caribbeans and Asians in Central Manchester. Br J Psychiatry 163:91–99, 1993

Tseng WS: Handbook of Cultural Psychiatry. San Diego, CA, Academic Press, 2001

Tseng WS, Matthews D, Elwyn T: Cultural Competency in Forensic Mental Health: Guide for Psychiatrists, Psychologists, and Attorneys. New York, Brunner-Routledge, 2004

Weinstein HC: Ethics issues in security hospitals. Behav Sci Law 20:443–461, 2002

Woon TH: The *latah* phenomenon. Oral presentation at the annual meeting of Pacific Rim College of Psychiatry, Hong Kong, 1988

Zhang XF: A report of 32 cases with hysteria involved in homicide [in Chinese]. Chinese Mental Health Journal 6(4):175–176, 1992

8

Culture and Child and Adolescent Psychiatry

S. Peter Kim, M.D., Ph.D., M.B.A.

Introduction: Culture and Children

Cultural Dimensions of Child Development

Child development has physical, cognitive, emotional, psychosocial, and environmental components that have a great deal of influence on developmental processes and outcomes. Although parents and family make up a major portion of a developing child's environment, their culture determines the values and mores that in turn mold the child's cultural orientation from very early in his or her development.

The physical growth and cognitive development of children across cultures follow genetic and hereditary transmission rules, which are based primarily on biological determinants. The emotional and psychosocial components of development are influenced by societal norms and traditions—namely, the culture in which the child is born and raised. Many aspects of that culture affect the continuum of the child's development. These include the cultural expectations of the birth (arrival) of a child; the meanings and values of a newborn child's biological and psychosocial attributes such as gender, birth order, and being born in or out of wedlock; child-rearing practices and the cultural significance attached to them; role expectations and role teachings of a child in different developmental stages; different values attached to child-rearing practice paradigms in various cultures; culturally appropriate behavioral norms of each developmental stage, according to the expected normal range of behavior in the culture; and determination of the child's psychosocial developmental norms in a culturally diverse and rapidly changing society such as the United States.

Ethnic identity develops parallel to ethnic socialization—the developmental processes by which children acquire the values, perceptions, behaviors, and attitudes of an ethnic group and perceive themselves and others as members of the group (Rotheram and Phinney 1986).

When a child is from a different culture, normal development and acculturation processes in the majority culture need to be understood according to a biopsychosocial paradigm, especially in determining the normalcy or pathology of each developmental stage, by highlighting the child's functional capability, adaptability, and malleability (Lee 1988). Parent-child conflicts, adolescent delinquency, and psychopathology in a transculturally migrated family may arise from the acculturation process. These occurrences should be carefully assessed, understood, and validated—on the basis of culturally sensitive and congruent assessment approaches—so that the clinician can make the most accurate and appropriate diagnosis, institute timely treatment interventions, and determine culturally appropriate long-term-care strategies when indicated.

Culture and Adolescents

Adolescence makes up its own unique culture in each of its developmental substages, with stage-specific tasks and a continuum of complex biological and psychosocial milestones and expectations to be attained for successful passage to adulthood. Adolescents with dual cultural heritages, from minority cultures, and from recent immigrant families from other cultures face acculturation tasks and adjustment to the majority culture. In addition, children from other cultures must go through the normal adolescent developmental tasks, eventually achieving the stage-specific psychosexual goal, "identity formation" or "consolidation of self-identity," that encompasses physical growth and cognitive development.

Some cultures encourage accelerated passage toward adulthood, with early rituals for manhood for boys and shortened adolescence. Cultures in Western technocratic societies tend to prolong adolescence with extended schooling and other educational and training periods. Across cultures, the common developmental tasks during adolescence are preparation for adulthood and identity formation.

Adolescents' intrapsychic conflicts and resultant anger and aggression are processed differently and to varying degrees in various cultures: for example, Western cultures tend to encourage sublimation through academic endeavors and physical sports, whereas traditional Confucian-influenced Asian cultures emphasize self-discipline, suppression, and self-refinement as the primary means of countering and resolving psychological conflicts and internal strife. Canino and Canino (1980) highlight aggression as a source of contention in Puerto Rican families who live in the mainland United States. Assertiveness, competitiveness, and independence—which are valued by American parents—contradict the core values of Puerto Rican culture. Strongly acculturated Puerto Rican children may be too assertive in the eyes of their parents.

Adolescents tend to respond to their conflicts through acting-out behavior that may lead to clinical pictures of conduct disorder. However, the tolerance thresholds of adults and the general public vary among different cultures. For example, in many Asian cultures the occasional group binge drinking of alcoholic beverages (although it may go beyond the ordinary ceremonial level) by late adolescents to celebrate certain individual or group events may be tolerated as the youths' way of sublimating their bottled-up energy or pressure. It is often viewed as the youngsters' preparation for self-mastery and control and a way "to expand the young ego" toward a healthy adulthood.

Although they are rapidly accepting Western—especially American—culture, most Asian and Far- and Mid-Eastern cultures still adhere to gender roles and segregate boys from girls, with adults' perception and criteria of sexual promiscuity being rather conservative and strict.

Culture and Parent-Child Relationships

Regardless of culture, children are perceived as being precious and in need of continuing nurturing and protection. In Western Judeo-Christian cultures, children are seen as God's gifts and as dependents to be protected and guided until they attain adulthood. The roles of parents are as guardians and protectors, with strong attachment being emphasized and appreciated. In traditional Chinese and other Asian cultures strongly influenced by Confucianism, hierarchical closeness, particularly between a father and his sons, is traditionally advocated and fostered, whereas the mother-daughter relationship is viewed as one of special closeness, warmth, and affection. In Japanese child-rearing practices, children are respected as special, independent individuals from a very early age. For example, parents use honorific forms of sentences when conversing with their young children. In most Asian cultures male children have traditionally been favored over female children, although that trend has been changing significantly over the past half century.

In families adjusting and adapting to a majority culture, such as recent immigrants to the United States, the relationship between parents and children is easily and frequently strained. Compared with the American host culture, most of the cultures from which these immigrant families come are conservative and place high values on parental authority, especially that of the father. Several psychosocial and cultural factors of these immigrant families tend to synergistically accelerate the development of intrafamily conflicts and friction between the children and their parents. These conflicts can result from the children's learning the language of the majority culture faster and better than their parents; the children's learning about the society and its cultural norms (and incorporating them) more readily than their parents; and the parents' feeling helpless under the pressure of adjusting to the new culture and perceiving themselves as unable to guide and control their children's behavior and adjustment processes. As a result of these conflicts, the parents may try to exert more authoritarian control over their children by rigidly imposing the values and codes of conduct of their original culture in a desperate attempt to maintain their authority as parents and guiding adults. Immigrant parents are often under tremendous pressure and can become frustrated in their acculturation processes, which are often slower and more difficult than their children's in many areas.

It has been reported that family discord or disruption influences a child's mental health more than socioeconomic status (Wolkind and Rutter 1985).

Case 1: A Boy Defies His Father at Home

David, a 15-year-old boy who is currently a freshman at an inner-city public high school in Los Angeles, immigrated to the United States from Thailand with his family when he was 8 years old. His father, a former high school principal in Bangkok, is currently running his own laundry, assisted by his wife. David is an only child. Despite initial difficulties in adjusting to the new culture, especially to his local public school class of predominantly Hispanic children, David has adjusted well to the school environment and has been an honor student since the fifth grade. He showed no behavioral problems until last year, when he began to defy his father's orders and his mother's advice. The emergence of this behavior coincided with the father's imposing an early curfew after learning that David was dating a Mexican American girl of his age, who is his classmate and is also an honor student.

The relationship between the father and the son rapidly deteriorated, and David's worsening defiant behavior culminated in his staying out overnight at his girlfriend's home without letting his parents know where he was. David's father, who had severe difficulties adjusting to the new culture, particularly with learning English, finally decided to see David's homeroom teacher and school counselor to find out what other serious problems David might be having in school. Through a family friend who was proficient in English, David's father learned that David had no behavior problems in school. Rather, he had consistently maintained his honor-roll status and was a role model for all his classmates. The father also learned that David had just been elected to represent his class in the student government.

Culture and Psychopathology of Children and Adolescents

There is no culture-specific psychopathology of children and adolescents. However, the level of understanding and acceptance of psychiatric disorders, tolerance of conduct problems, and perception and concepts of psychopathology of children and adolescents vary among people from different cultural environments.

Child Neglect/Abuse and Sexual Abuse

Abuse of children of any kind, whether neglect or physical or sexual abuse, reflects the incompetence of the parents or caretakers of the victimized child. By definition, *neglect* is withholding or inadequate provision of the child's basic physical and emotional needs for his or her normal and healthy development. *Abuse* involves physical and emotional harm done to the child, whether or not the harm is irreversible. *Sexual abuse* includes any kind of sexual assault of the child; it often traumatizes the child physically as well as emotionally, leaving, in most instances, permanent scars on the victim's psyche and leading to developmental, behavioral, or emotional disorders.

In all contemporary societies and cultures around the world, any form of neglect or abuse of children that harms their normal developmental progresses is illegal and condemned. However, child abuse occurs mostly as a result of parental psychopathology, often associated with family environments of socioeconomic disadvantage, reflecting social and environmental factors that are conducive to fostering the child's developmental vulnerabilities. Parents or caretakers of abused children often have mental disorders or substance abuse disorders.

In some cultures, corporal punishment has traditionally been accepted and used as a disciplinary or corrective measure for conduct disorders in children and adolescents. When such culturally sanctioned disciplinary measures continue to be practiced by immigrant families in a new, majority Western culture—especially the United States—they may constitute blatant child abuse. The practices are deemed to incur physical and emotional damage in the child and are prohibited by law. Often ignorance on the immigrant parents' part leads them to serious trouble with child-protection and other concerned government agencies for violating child-protection laws.

Conduct Disorders

In the United States, statutory mandates are clearly spelled out in the law and are enforced for the protection of children to prevent them from becoming delinquent and negligent in their schoolwork. However, few developing countries have statutory guidelines stipulating and enforcing minors' conduct. Also, the DSM-IV-TR (American Psychiatric Association 2000) diagnostic criteria for conduct disorder include violations of statutory mandates for minors, such as curfew violations, unauthorized school absenteeism, and running away from home. Although some Asian and European cultures place a high value on school education, self-discipline, and responsibility, other (mainly agricultural) societies tend to place less importance on regular school attendance and strict enforcement of the codes of conduct for minors.

It has been commonly reported that conduct disorders among children and adolescents have a high negative correlation with parental supervision, family stability, and parental socioeconomic status. Many recent immigrant families experience multiple difficulties: parental difficulties in adjusting to the new society, including learning the new language; finding a job to support the family; and ensuring that their children are properly educated and encounter as few difficulties as possible in adjusting to the new culture.

When family stability is not secured and intrafamily stress and tension are high, parents are likely to fail to maintain the lines of communication with their children. This fundamental breakdown in the family security system can contribute to a child's drifting toward delinquency. Lack of understanding and awareness of the new society and its culture render parents unable to supervise their children to ensure that they acquire the expected behavioral norms of the new society.

In evaluating minority youngsters, especially those from the inner city, it is crucial to obtain information on the family and neighborhood

(Canino and Spurlock 1994). Often there is a history of child abuse or neglect. It is essential to ask about the possibility of lead poisoning and malnutrition. Other predisposing factors to disruptive behavior disorders in children and adolescents include parental abuse of alcohol and other substances and antisocial personality disorder in a family member.

People from some (principally agricultural) cultures tend to place less importance on the disciplinary aspects of child rearing and guiding the conduct of their adolescents. Parents with these cultural backgrounds tend to have a higher tolerance for certain negative behavior patterns in their children that might be viewed as deviant and delinquent according to the behavioral norms and standards of most developed Western cultures.

Eating Disorders and Obesity

In many cases, eating disorders are related to cultural and subcultural factors in culinary-oriented families. In most Asian cultures in the past, a large physique and an obese body were viewed as signs of a person's financial prosperity and prominent social status, showing that the person was able to afford an abundance of high-calorie food. In some family subcultures, cooking is the major collective family activity and the center of the family's happiness and pleasure. Whenever they have an opportunity, all the family members gather to cook and share the joys of having a big meal together.

Despite the accumulating modern medical knowledge that obesity is a threat to one's physical health and may also be either the cause or the result of psychological problems, people of certain minority cultures or subcultures persist in their unhealthy eating habits.

The psychodynamics and psychopathogenesis of eating disorders and obesity in children and adolescents remain almost identical across various cultures and countries.

Hyperactive Behavior and a Spectrum of Related Disorders

The terms *hyperactivity* and *hyperkinesis* have been used frequently to connote a clinical syndrome of attention-deficit/hyperactivity disorder (ADHD). Before making a conclusive psychiatric diagnosis of ADHD according to DSM-IV-TR criteria, a clinician must carefully take into consideration all the possible contributing factors that might have affected the child whose behavioral symptoms mimic the symptoms and signs of ADHD. These include the presence of anxiety disorder, psychosocial and educational pressure, worries and fears arising from peer conflicts, intrafamily conflicts (particularly parental disharmony), excessive intake of stimulants (such as caffeine-containing beverages), and a high activity level (or simply always being cheerful and full of energy).

Cultural factors contribute significantly to the perception, acceptance, treatment, and management of ADHD. The wide range in incidence and prevalence rates of ADHD across nations and cultures indicates differing views about the management of a hyperactive or highly active child. Also, the level of tolerance by the major caretaker of a child's highly active behavior—including that of a child with diagnostically confirmed ADHD—varies among different socioeconomic, cultural, and ethnic groups. A highly active preschool-age boy who is always in motion, running around his 3-acre yard and six-bedroom home in an affluent suburban community, may be viewed by his parents and neighbors as simply a very energetic boy. However, a boy of the same age and high activity level of minority ethnicity, with a single mother and five siblings living in a crowded two-bedroom walk-up apartment in a public housing project in an inner city area, may not be fondly accepted by his mother and neighbors. Often such children from families in lower socioeconomic levels are forced to go to a children's mental health clinic for a diagnostic evaluation. Statistics indicate that ADHD is three to seven times more prevalent among elementary school children of lower socioeconomic and ethnic-minority communities than among middle-class and upper-middle-class communities in the United States. Many factors that can adversely affect a child's prenatal, perinatal, and postnatal development are directly and indirectly associated with ADHD and other developmental disorders, including learning and language disorders. These adverse prenatal and perinatal factors, to name just a few, include poor maternal health during pregnancy; maternal abuse of legal or illegal medications (such as alcohol, marijuana, and other prescription drugs) during pregnancy; poor and inadequate prenatal (maternal and fetal) health care; malnutrition; maternal illnesses or surgical procedures under general anesthesia during pregnancy; difficult and prolonged labor; jaundice; birth trauma to the child; and frequent infections of the baby, such as in seizure disorder.

Case 2: A Boy Who Was Fidgety

José, a 6-year-old second grader who had been in America for just over 2 years, had immigrated from El Salvador with his family, which con-

sisted of José, his parents, and two older siblings. The father was a political refugee who had been a senior civil engineer in an important,
high-level position. Now he was working as a live-in manager of an old
apartment building, where the family lived. José's parents were having
a difficult time adjusting to the new culture, especially learning English.
José's teachers found him to be always fidgety, constantly looking
around, squeezing his hands, and not concentrating on his classroom
work. About 1 month into the new semester he was referred to a community children's mental health clinic for diagnostic evaluation to rule
ADHD in or out and for appropriate treatment and management advice. The clinic's child psychiatrist found José to be a bright and energetic boy who was able to pay attention appropriately and as directed
but remained tense throughout the evaluation session and appeared to
be afraid of something. A physical examination and other screening
tests did not reveal any soft neurological signs of attention difficulties.
However, José volunteered that he had been drinking two to three cups
of Colombian coffee every morning before he left for school in an effort
to stay awake in the classroom and that his parents always drank several cups of coffee at breakfast and many more during the rest of the
day. José had been having nightmares and also was very worried about
his parents, who were having increasingly frequent, severe arguments,
with both recently threatening to leave home. The diagnoses were childhood anxiety disorder with caffeine-induced high vigilance and hyperactivity and moderate to severe adjustment reaction.

Teenage Substance Abuse

During the past several decades, abuse of illicit drugs among adolescents and youths has become a rising major social, developmental, educational, and public health concern throughout the United States and
in developed and developing countries all over the world. Several factors have been suggested as contributing to illicit substance abuse, leading many abusers to dependence, especially during adolescence and
young adulthood: biological vulnerabilities, including low pain thresh-
old; a genetic predisposition to dependency; socioeconomic vulnerabilities, such as living in a drug-culture environment; the presence of
criminally inclined peers and adult role models; financial pressure and
temptation to be pulled into drug dealings; curiosity and peer pressure
to partake in the use of drugs; psychological vulnerabilities, such as depression, bipolar affective disorder, and other major psychiatric disorders that lower self-control or compromise one's sound judgment
capacity; identity confusion or crisis, desperation, and eventual self-
abandonment.

Most youths who abuse illicit drugs tend to come from single-parent
families of lower socioeconomic classes and to have had inadequate or

no parental supervision. Often these substance-abusing youngsters report a history of parental substance abuse or drug-related criminal offenses, for which their parents have been or are currently incarcerated in a state or federal penitentiary.

The environment in a subculture of drug abuse taints the developmental processes of these adolescents and youths with distorted value systems and justifications or rationalizations for the illegal acts committed around them and by them as the lifestyle model after which to pattern themselves.

Children from traditional, conservative cultures that accept and maintain a hierarchical family and social structure (such as traditional Asian and Latino cultures) tend to have a lower incidence of substance abuse, provided their families remain intact and they have ongoing parental—especially paternal—supervision. The fathers provide role models of positive values and ideals, which, although based on their cultures of origin, are steadily and consistently upheld and instilled in their children. The adolescents and youths who have abused or have become dependent on illegal substances have a high incidence of dual psychiatric diagnoses and may concurrently have conditions such as chronic depression, anxiety disorders (including posttraumatic stress disorder or panic disorder), major depression, bipolar affective disorder, and ADHD (with or without a learning disorder).

Other Psychopathologies in Cultural Contexts

It has been reported that there is a high incidence of paranoia or paranoid disorder among immigrant populations. The impact of such psychopathology on a child's development and on the psychopathogenesis of childhood-onset mental disorders has not been adequately or systematically studied. Immigrant parents who have just moved to the United States tend to be more restrictive of their children's behavior and excessively concerned about their welfare, safety, and success. These parental attitudes and attempts to control their children's lives often lead to resistance or open rebelliousness from the children (particularly teenage children), which may further aggravate the already strained child-parent relationship. The worst outcome is a total cessation of communication between the parents and their children, which is the major cause among adolescents and youths of acting-out behavior, depression, and full-blown behavioral manifestations of juvenile delinquency.

Culturally Competent Assessment of Children and Adolescents

A clinician who evaluates children and adolescents of different or diverse cultural backgrounds should have a good understanding of their evaluees' original cultures and other culture-related issues that have influenced all areas of their developmental processes. Contrary to earlier contentions of scholars and clinicians in the field, the evaluating clinician does not necessarily have to be of the same ethnic or cultural background as the child. The clinician may be culturally competent as long as he or she has a good working knowledge of the child's culture of origin, adequate clinical skills, empathy and a willingness to work with the child and his or her family, and a continuing interest in learning more about the child and his or her culture.

Psychiatric Assessments

The clinician evaluating a child from a different or minority culture must be aware of and understand the parents' perception of psychiatry and mental health evaluation in the context of their original culture. The clinician must be sensitive, skillful, and resourceful enough in dealing with the parents' needs and desires to secure their commitment to participate actively in the evaluation and treatment of the child.

In many Asian and Hispanic cultures, children are viewed as belonging to and dependent on their parents. Children are expected to be obedient and subordinate to parental authority. Therefore, the autonomy and independence of children are not recognized or emphasized as much as they are in some other cultures, such as contemporary Euro-American cultures. Rather, allowing children and adolescents their autonomy and independence before they reach an appropriate age is often viewed in these cultures as abandoning the parental obligation and duty of caring for the youngsters.

In most situations, except for emergencies, it is advised that the clinician first see the parents alone, without the child, in order to explain the purposes and benefits of the evaluation and to assess the degree of parental understanding and awareness of the child's emotional and behavioral difficulties. This fact-finding interview will also allow the parents to ask any questions they might have about the child as well as the evaluation itself and to share family issues and history that they believe might be helpful for the clinician. This interview with the parents also reinforces parental authority and helps align the parents as allies in the evaluation and treatment processes.

In Asian cultures mental illness or behavioral problems have traditionally been viewed as personal and social stigmata that bring shame to the affected individual and to the whole family. When, in desperation, families of psychiatric patients have sought outside help from a mental health professional under pressure from either a government agency (e.g., social services, school, or family court) or close family friends, it usually means that the psychiatric condition of the affected family member is serious and beyond the family's ability and resources to deal with. Most ethnic-minority or immigrant families in such crisis situations have already gone through all available alternative treatments—including traditional herb medicine, folk healing or rituals such as exorcism rites, and other culture-specific traditional remedies. The examining psychiatrist should understand the cultural aspects of mental illness—such as the dynamics arising from the mental illness in the patient's traditional, hierarchical family constellation—and the family's initial views and expectations of Western medical and psychiatric specialists. The psychiatrist should respect and display empathy toward the family, offering gentle and thorough explanations and guidance on the nature and prognosis of the mental illness that their loved one is experiencing. It is important to invite the family members to be therapeutic allies and partners in the treatment process from the very beginning of the strategic planning stage.

The family should be continuously and repeatedly reminded of its partnership with the psychiatrist or treatment team. This trusting relationship should be consolidated and maintained through ongoing, open, candid communications.

Sufficient time should be allocated to the family interview sessions for the interpretation of the primary language of the family and for the complete and thorough collection of pertinent historical data about the patient, past illnesses, and family history, as well as past treatment history, modalities, and methods. The family should be given the option of designating a family member, either the most senior or the senior's designee, as a contact person or spokesperson to work with the treating psychiatrist and the treatment team to facilitate timely communication of information between the two parties.

Psychometric Assessments

The purpose, nature, and benefits of psychometric tests to be administered to the child or adolescent patient should be carefully and thoroughly explained to the patient and the family, and appropriate informed consent should be obtained well in advance of test administration.

Because almost no psychometric tests have been proved to be culture neutral, every effort must be made to secure a culturally sensitive and bilingual tester and culturally standardized or culture-sensitive test materials (Cattell 1959). The results should be interpreted with careful consideration of the patient's linguistic proficiency in the test language, familiarity with the test materials in his or her cultural context, degree and congruence of performance inhibition relative to the behavioral norms in his or her primary culture, and degree of acculturation.

Many leading psychometricians have attempted to develop culture-neutral and universally applicable tests that can be used for children and adolescents across cultures, but results have been far from satisfactory to both the researchers and test subjects. Although there is a general consensus among psychometricians and test subjects on the impossibility of devising psychometric tests that are absolutely culture neutral, the degree of cultural biases can be minimized or correctively adjusted in scoring to maximize internal consistency and obtain a true, valid cognitive projective profile of the test subject. It has been emphasized that the test results merely reflect the test subject's cognitive and personality profile at a given point in time and under the unique circumstances of the test. This reminds the interpreter and users of the test results of the importance of test-retest comparison and consistency as well as cultural influences.

The linguistic proficiency and competence of the test subject in the language of the test materials have considerable effects on the test results because they affect the degree of understanding of the test questions or tasks and the test subject's ability to respond accurately to the test stimuli. Cultural interpretations of certain objects and behavior, as well as culturally instilled values and culture-prescribed idiosyncratic interpretations thereof, all affect the way the test subject cognitively and behaviorally responds to the test stimuli.

Case 3: A Boy Suspected of Having Cognitive Deficits

Pedro, an 8-year-old Hispanic boy and a third grader in a local public school, was referred for a cognitive psychometric test to determine if he had any cognitive deficits, namely, the features of mental retardation. Pedro and his family had come to the United States as immigrants from Nicaragua, in Central America, about 2 years previously. Pedro's father had been a high-ranking government official in the Nicaraguan Central Bank, and both of his parents were college graduates with traditional, conservative upbringings. Pedro's teachers felt that Pedro was a nice boy who always tried hard to please his teachers and classmates, but he appeared to be slow in learning. He always remained quiet and never verbally expressed himself in the classroom except when asked by the teacher. The tests were administered by a bilingual clinician-tester in both English and Spanish. The results indicated that Pedro's overall intelligence was above his age norm. However, Pedro remained very passive, but compliant, throughout the session, never taking any initiative and only saying things or doing tasks that were specifically asked of him by the tester, an authority figure. The examiner found that Pedro had been taught by his parents from early in his childhood that a boy of "good" conduct does not say anything in the presence of elders or authority figures, such as a father, an elderly person, doctors, or teachers, unless he is invited to verbally express his thoughts and ideas. It was also found that Pedro readily recognized and named a guitar, but not a violin, because the latter musical instrument was not common in his experiences in Nicaragua.

Other Considerations in Assessment of a Child From Another Culture

In assessing a child of a different cultural background clinically and by psychometric tests, the examining mental health professional should be mindful of several basic, essential issues that have contributed to the child's emotional and cognitive development. In the following paragraphs we outline a few areas in which the child's past cultural environment can have a great deal of influence.

Cultural Attitudes and Upbringing of a Child

In most cultures, children are viewed as the hope of the future and the bearers of cultural values and national pride and heritage. However, there are differences in the way the child is viewed from adult and parental perspectives. In most Asian and Latino cultures, children are viewed as helpless individuals who are dependent on adults and need constant nurturing, support, and protection. In Japanese culture, although children's dependence is recognized, they are given a degree of respect equal to that shown to adults, such as parental usage of honorific words and teaching the children to respect individuals of all ages equally. In Mexican culture, generosity, mutual support, and reciprocal assistance are often valued (Kunce and Vales 1984).

In Western cultures, especially Anglo-American culture, emphasis is placed on assertiveness, outspokenness, individualism, and independence from the very earliest phases of child rearing. This is demonstrated in the sleeping arrangements of a child. In American and most Western cultures, it is common for the child to have his or her own separate room from an early age. In Asian, Latino, and some African cultures, many children still sleep in the same bedroom as their parents, or in a room adjacent to the parents' room, until the beginning of elementary school. In many Asian societies that are under the influence of Confucianism, children and women are subordinate to the father or male head of the family, who guides and protects them in all areas.

Hierarchical and Horizontal Authority Structures

The hierarchical structure of authority in the family and the society influence a child's upbringing, concept formation and attitudes toward authority figures, and development of inner codes of conduct in relationship to them. Children from the hierarchical authority-oriented societies of Asian regions learn from early in their development that adults and authority figures are to be shown absolute respect and unquestioning obedience. No challenge, verbal or nonverbal, toward these figures is acceptable. Most children who come to the United States from such cultures are quiet and taciturn in their classes beyond a reasonable adjustment period. This behavior causes their teachers to question whether they have been intellectually compromised for earlier medical or other reasons, are emotionally disturbed, or both (see "Case 3: A Boy Suspected of Having Cognitive Deficits" above).

Culture, Learning, and Experiential Differences

Each culture has its own unique, idiosyncratic ways of determining priorities in children's educational and learning experiences. In Western (primarily technocratic) cultures, emphasis is placed on the development of skills and knowledge needed for success in the individual's professional and vocational career, mostly measured by monetary success and fame.

In Eastern cultures, particularly in Eastern Asia, individual success is traditionally measured by how high a position one can attain in the governmental or public-service hierarchy, which gives one recognized authority and honor. Historically, to be appointed to such prestigious positions, one had to pass extremely arduous and competitive government-monitored national examinations, often under the direct auspices of the king (or, in modern times, the head of the government). Hence, the education of a child is a top priority among parents.

In such cultures, teachers or other professionals with a teacher's attributes in their titles or professional positions are given absolute respect and obedience. This is also in keeping with the highest Confucian teaching that a man must submit to and respect three unchallengeable entities in life: the king, the father, and teachers.

Cultural Aspects of Mental Health Care of Children and Adolescents

In this section, psychiatric treatments and related general mental health services are reviewed from cultural perspectives. Essential guidelines for the treatment of children and families from different cultures are presented, along with suggestions on working with ethnic minorities and families of different cultural backgrounds and ways to implement culturally appropriate, competent treatment modalities.

Essential Guidelines

Psychiatric disorders and patients with mental illnesses are still viewed with biases even in the most medically rational, socially accommodating, liberal, egalitarian, modern societies, such as the United States. In most cultures and countries with traditional, conservative values, psychiatric disorders are not well or correctly understood or accepted as one category of medical malady among all human medical illnesses. In almost all developing societies, most people with mental illnesses (or their families) anxiously seek professional help. However, they are cautious and fearful lest they be stigmatized or discriminated against because of their mental illness or the mental illness of a family member. Despite these inhibiting social and cultural forces, they often reach a point of desperation that forces them to seek professional psychiatric help because mental health treatment resources are either inadequate or unavailable within their traditional communities.

When a family head or parent from such a cultural background consults with a mental health professional about a family member who has been experiencing a mental illness, the elder is either having serious problems managing the patient, whose psychiatric symptoms and behavior are on the verge of being out of control, or has exhausted all other available alternative means of treatment. The parents or family elder are beyond the point of caring about saving face and family dignity from the stigma of being known among neighbors and friends as the family of a psychiatrically ill patient or, worse, as a "mental illness family." The consulting psychiatrist and mental health team must be sensitive to the family members' anxiety, concerns, fear, shame, and guilt. Respect and empathy should be extended to them, and every effort should be made to make them feel cared for, comfortable, and dignified.

It is important to give the family elders, parents of the patient, or legal guardians an opportunity to discuss the patient before the patient is seen, even in a crisis situation, in order to give them a sense of control and respect. This will in turn help lay the foundation for a better therapeutic alliance for the period of treatment.

The treating psychiatrist should keep the family and parents closely informed of the treatment progress of the patient to the extent permitted by the physician's time, ethical guidelines, and laws protecting patient information.

In most cultures in developing societies, particularly in Asian and Latino societies, physicians are viewed as important authority figures. The patients' families are cautiously respectful of them and tend to try not to bother them by calling them, although they may have many medical and other patient-related questions for which they want answers or explanations. Hence, it is important for the treating psychiatrist to tell the parents that it is all right and even encouraged for them to call and ask whatever questions they may have regarding the patient's illness and prognosis, the kind and nature of treatments being implemented, and the overall progress of the patient.

In the case of inpatient treatment, the patient's and family's desires to incorporate their culture-specific lifestyle or customs into the overall treatment plans, from dress to meal habits, should be accommodated as far as hospital rules and local laws permit.

In summary, the essentials for mental health professionals to successfully help culturally diversified children and adolescent patients and their families are to be sensitive to the patient's culture and customs and to accommodate and incorporate them constructively into the treatment plan and implementation.

Working With the Family

The family is the most important environment and support system for a child's healthy growth and development. In the treatment of mental health or behavioral problems of a child or adolescent, particularly of a different cultural background, working with the family is the first step in securing a helpful therapeutic alliance and creating a therapeutically conducive treatment environment. When a child is in need of mental health treatment, parents are under the dual stress of trying to grasp the true nature of the child's illness and assisting the child and the treatment team in making the treatment process expedient and successful. Regardless of the cultural background of the family, the majority of parents of children in need of psychiatric help must deal with fear, shame, and guilt along with denial and minimization of the child's emotional, cognitive, or behavioral condition.

In most minority families, the father is at the top of the family hierarchy and needs to be treated with respect and deference by the treatment team. The mother, in most cases, is in charge of the close supervision of the child. She is the main caretaker, providing all of the child's developmental and basic physical needs, including food and clothing, and assisting in the child's extracurricular activities, such as socializing with friends and other adults. In middle-class, majority communities in the United States, it is primarily the mothers who oversee the children's school activities and supervise their homework during elementary school and high school.

It is also very important for the treating psychiatrist to help maintain the dignity and authority of recently migrated or ethnic-minority parents (especially fathers) in the presence of the child patient and other siblings, such as during an intake interview or while conducting a family session to gather information about the family. Any issues that may have to do with parental shortcomings or mistakes should be postponed until a later information session between the parents and the psychiatrist, without the children.

When the parents' lack of English proficiency requires an interpreter, it is best to arrange to have a competent, professional interpreter who is from the same ethnic and cultural background as the family, rather than relying on the bilingual child or adolescent patient to serve as an interpreter between the therapist and the parents. Using the child or adolescent patient as an interpreter risks compromising parental dignity and distorting information needed for diagnostic and therapeutic purposes.

Culturally Sensitive Treatment Approaches

Canino and Spurlock (1994) emphasize that treatment facilities for children from culturally diverse backgrounds must be accessible and provide comprehensive and culturally sensitive services. A study by Rogler and colleagues (1985) suggests three ways of rendering mental health services that are culturally sensitive to ethnocultural minority populations: increase accessibility to psychotherapy by locating mental health clinics in minority neighborhoods and close to public transportation; employ mental health workers who share the linguistic and cultural backgrounds of the patients; and create an ambience that reflects the cultural heritage of the client population.

In treating a child and family from a culture that is different from the majority culture of the United States, the therapist's sensitivity, understanding, and knowledge of the patient's culture are essential prerequisites to treatment. Empathy and willingness to help the needy minority child and adolescent populations are important but are not the most essential components for successful treatment.

The importance of clinician variables in treating minority populations has been discussed from cross-cultural mental health service perspectives. These variables, difficult but not impossible to assess, most likely exert a greater impact on the success or failure of treatment strategies with children than with adults. The clinician's age, sex, and ethnicity, in addition to his or her empathic and perceptive skills, emerge as factors that need to balance well with his or her theoretical orientation and ability to interact and communicate with children of various ethnic and cultural backgrounds. The clinician who works with children must be straightforward and honest, intellectually curious and flexible, and emotionally able to deal with the psychological challenges of younger patients (Canino and Spurlock 1994).

It is important to note that in many cultures in developing societies—notably in Asia, South America, and Africa—parents and relatives of mentally ill children and adolescents tend to seek treatment relief and support from outside the modern mental health system. To serve the families of mentally ill patients who are unable to heal within these unconventional, traditional healing networks, mental health professionals must penetrate the lay referral structure by assimilating some members of the ethnic network into the professional structure. It has been suggested that a client's initial registration at a mental health facility should be informal and immediate (Flores 1978).

In addition to the cultural sensitivity of the treating professional, a well-selected and well-organized multidisciplinary team plays a crucial role in a successful treatment outcome. The members of the team should continually try to improve their treatment skills, along with enhancing their cultural sensitivity and knowledge through formal and informal education and training built into the team as an essential program component.

Medication and Ethnicity

It has been generally accepted among psychiatric clinicians that certain ethnic groups are more sensitive to psychotropic medications than others. For example, Chinese, Korean, and Japanese patients tend to require much lower medication doses, at times as little as half or one-third of the doses required by Caucasian patients. The currently accepted view is that genetic factors may explain not only interindividual but also cross-ethnic variations in drug responses (Lin et al. 1993).

The therapeutic dosages of most psychotropic medications for children under age 12 have not been well established, even for those of Caucasian descent. It has been cautioned that psychotropic medications should be administered to children under 12 more conservatively in dosage and duration, because long-term developmental, psychological, and behavioral complications—including effects on physical growth and psychological and cognitive development, and adverse behavioral effects leading to substance abuse—have not been well researched or understood.

The ethnic differences in children's responses to psychotropic medications, such as pharmacodynamics and pharmacokinetics, are not completely known. Much more needs to be learned in these areas in future clinical and biological research.

It is still controversial whether doses of psychotropic medications for children should be above or below the dose per kilogram body weight equivalent recommended for adults. One camp insists that the doses should be adjusted to much higher levels because the hepatic metabolic rates of children and adolescents are much higher than those in adults. Another camp warns that it is not the dose but the combination of pharmacokinetics and individual neurophysiological sensitivity to drugs—including ethnicity-specific sensitivity—that matters.

References

American Psychiatric Association: Diagnostic and Statistical Manual of Mental Disorders, 4th Edition, Text Revision. Washington, DC, American Psychiatric Association, 2000

Canino IA, Canino G: Impact of stress on the Puerto Rican family: treatment considerations. Am J Orthopsychiatry 50:535–541, 1980

Canino IA, Spurlock J: Culturally Diverse Children and Adolescents: Assessment, Diagnosis and Treatment. New York, Guilford, 1994

Cattell RB: Handbook for the Culture Fair Intelligence Test: A Measure of "G." Champaign, IL, Institute for Personality and Ability Testing, 1959

Flores JL: The utilization of a community mental health service by Mexican-Americans. Int J Soc Psychiatry 24:271–275, 1978

Kunce JT, Vales LF: The Mexican American: implications for cross-cultural rehabilitation counseling. Rehabil Couns Bull 28:97–108, 1984

Lee E: Cultural factors in working with Southeast Asian refugee adolescents. J Adolesc 11:167–179, 1988

Lin KM, Poland RE, Nakasaki G (eds): Psychopharmacology and Psychobiology of Ethnicity. Washington, DC, American Psychiatric Press, 1993

Rogler LH, Blumenthal R, Malgady R, et al: Hispanics and Culturally Sensitive Mental Health Services. (Research Bulletin 8). New York, Fordham University, Hispanic Research Center, 1985

Rotheram MJ, Phinney JS: Introduction: definitions and perspectives in the study of children's ethnic socialization, in Children's Ethnic Socialization: Pluralism and Development. Edited by Phinney JS, Rotheram MJ. Newbury Park, CA, Sage, 1986, pp 10–28

Wolkind S, Rutter M: Sociocultural Factors in Child and Adolescent Psychiatry. Boston, MA, Blackwell Scientific, 1985

9

Culture and Geriatric Psychiatry

Junji Takeshita, M.D.
Iqbal Ahmed, M.D.

Introduction: Culture and Aging

Becoming old is a natural part of life. How each individual deals with the aging process is influenced by a number of factors, and significantly so by premorbid personality styles. Short of a personality change due to a medical disorder, it is doubtful that a pessimistic, introverted middle-aged person will suddenly become optimistic and extroverted with old age. The cultural background of an individual also plays a major role in determining how the aging process is viewed. Indeed, growing old in a Western culture is often seen as something to be avoided and feared. Youth is highly valued, and the appearance of aging is put off as much as possible. Staggering amounts of money are spent on "anti-aging" creams, plastic surgeries, and other treatments. Becoming old in Western societies is typically associated with social isolation, disability, and inevitable placement in a nursing home. On the other hand, some non-Western societies associate the elderly with wisdom and knowledge. Understandably, in such cultures the aging process is not feared and may even be welcomed.

The percentage increase in the number of elderly persons worldwide is enormous, and this is true in the United States population as well. This growth has been particularly dramatic among the ethnic-minority elderly in the United States. The ethnic-minority population is currently about 17% of the United States population, and by 2050 it will have increased to 36% (U.S. Administration on Aging 2003). Japan now has mandatory long-term-care insurance to deal with aging (Chiarolanza 2001). In developing countries such as China, life span has increased dramatically, resulting in significant social changes.

The role of culture in the aging process, unfortunately, is not simple. With technological and scientific developments such as telecommunication, and with increasing globalization, it is too simplistic to think in terms of Western and non-Western. Nursing homes are a growing industry in Japan, a country typically associated with reverence for the elderly. In the United States, there are elderly of many ethnic cultures, both minority and Caucasian. Each minority group has pertinent historical experiences (Baker and Lightfoot 1993). For example, Native American groups were victims of genocide and have a history of forced attendance in boarding schools where speaking in their native language was punished, whereas African Americans have endured a legacy of slavery and legalized segregation. Even within each minority group there is considerable heterogeneity. For example, a recently arrived African elderly person with no command of English has relatively little in common with an African American elderly individual whose ancestors were brought to the continent as slaves. In fact, due to variations in life experiences, there is greater heterogeneity among the elderly than among younger cohorts. Therefore, in consideration of the effects of culture and aging on psychopathology and treatment, the specific cohort experience may in fact be a key variable.

Not surprisingly, the elderly groups of all cultures have been low utilizers of mental health services. New immigrant elderly persons are especially unlikely to seek mental health treatment, although the need may be greater among this group and their family resources are often limited. In this chapter we discuss evaluation and treatment considerations for dealing with culture in the elderly.

Definition of Aging

Aging is obviously a universal process, but there is no consistency among cultures regarding what age is considered old. Typically, *old* is defined by external factors, such as retirement and receipt of Social Security benefits. There do appear to be ethnic differences in what is considered old (Freed 1992). Mexican Americans defined themselves as old at 57 years on average; African Americans, at 63 years; and Caucasian Americans, at 70 years. Members of minority groups may feel old due to hardship, typically financial in nature. For example, Caucasian

Americans, African Americans, and Mexican Americans all stated that the biggest problem with aging was finance. For African Americans the second biggest worry was crime, and for Mexican Americans it was the cost of food. For Caucasian American elderly persons the second biggest problem was isolation and loneliness, reflecting the seriousness of a psychosocial problem.

There may be differing norms regarding age-appropriate behavior, as well as what is considered to be healthy aging (Fry 1988). There also may be formal staging or ceremonies to identify transitions that, in most cultures, assist in the healthy adaptation to aging. However, there may be cultural variations in what is considered healthy aging. Disengagement, continuity, or active engagement in society may each be the norm of healthy aging in different cultures. There also may be some universal norms or patterns of aging, especially with regard to gender differences in aging (Guttman 1975). Women move from passive to active mastery and men from active to passive mastery. In other words, men and women tend to become more alike as they age. This may be due to sociocultural views of gender roles or, more likely, biological changes such as alterations in the endocrine function of testosterone and estrogen.

Acculturation Issues

Acculturation is an easier process for a younger person, and the differences in acculturation between the generations may have negative influences on the psychological well-being of members of the older generation (Markides et al. 1990). The elderly individual has a language barrier that leads to less interaction with the majority culture. There may be little need to speak or learn English. Meanwhile, the younger generation has acculturated with the majority culture through work and social interactions. Thus, the elderly individual has expectations that are not congruent with those of the younger members of the family. All families have such a "generation gap," but such differences are increased with differences in acculturation. Immigrant elderly persons may cling to old values from the home country, even through the home country has evolved as well (Gelfand 1994). For example, even in Japan there has been a rapid breakdown of the extended family, a concept virtually unthinkable a generation previously.

Family and Intergenerational Issues

There may be cultural influences on issues such as filial responsibility, filial piety, familialism (the tendency to keep family issues away from outsiders), and dependence of elders on children and grandchildren. As an effect of acculturation, differing expectations of younger and older group members may result in conflict between the adopted culture and the native culture. To resolve these conflicts, there has to be negotiation among the family members and ultimately an accommodation (Ahmed 1997).

Attitudes About Widowhood, Grief, and Bereavement

In the United States, most women marry older men, yet women have a longer life span. Thus, women typically have a longer period of widowed life (Zisook and Shuchter 1996). The roles of the widow and widower are different in many cultures. For example, in India a widow cannot remarry, but a widower can. Widowers may have different issues, compared with widows. Japanese and Korean men typically do not help with domestic chores. As a result, widowers from such countries have a difficult time coping with such chores as cooking. Chinese men, on the other hand, frequently assist in the kitchen, and such tasks are therefore less of a problem after the death of a spouse.

Attitudes Toward Nursing Homes

Nursing homes are common in Western cultures and reflect a practical solution to caring for large numbers of debilitated elderly persons who require custodial-level nursing care. The framework of a nuclear family does not allow for practical care of large numbers of elderly individuals. In many non-Western cultures, the emphasis on extended families and the proportionately smaller elderly population (due to shorter life spans) often allow for home care of the ill elderly. Obviously, this poses a significant problem in developing countries that are rapidly becoming Westernized. In addition, elderly immigrants to Western countries are disappointed by the values of their Westernized children, daughters-in-law, sons-in-law, and grandchildren, who may be very comfortable with the idea of nursing home placement.

Death

Death is the inevitable outcome of the aging process. In the United States, many elderly persons of all ethnic groups die in the hospital, but in other countries, such as Samoa, death is treated as a natural part of the life process, not requiring special care. Even Western poems dealing with death have alluded to the need to struggle against it (e.g., "Do

Not Go Gentle Into That Good Night" by Dylan Thomas [1952]). This probably again reflects death anxiety and emphasis on youth culture. Preparation for death also involves issues of religion, whether Christian, Buddhist, Muslim, or other faiths (Braun et al. 2000). Advanced directives, living wills, and surrogate decision making are all parts of the process of death and dying in the United States. The medicolegal system in Western countries is often at odds with the natural process of dying.

Culturally Influenced Psychopathology

Depression

The DSM-IV-TR (American Psychiatric Association 2000) diagnostic criteria for major depression are the same for all patients, regardless of age or culture. For example, somatic symptoms and anxiety tend to be more prevalent in elderly persons, but such symptoms are not included in the DSM-IV-TR diagnosis. Ethnic-minority elders may particularly use somatic symptoms. They may prefer to complain of a headache or feeling dizzy, rather than acknowledge sadness or depression (Sakauye 1996). Ethnic-minority elders who are new to the country, having spent most of their productive years elsewhere, are at greater risk for depression when they move into communities without peers or ethnic-community supports, such as churches. Issues such as minority status, discrimination, and socioeconomic status may be additional risk factors for depression and other psychiatric problems.

Suicide

Compared with the general elderly population, ethnic-minority elderly persons tend to have lower rates of completed suicide, with the possible exception of Chinese Americans and Japanese Americans older than age 75 (Baker 1994). This may reflect a cohort effect. Immigration laws in the early part of the twentieth century did not allow for Chinese men to bring their families into the country. As a result, many Chinese men are now old and alone without any family support. Suicide rates among Japanese elderly men are not dramatically different from those in the Caucasian population. However, the factors influencing suicide in these groups may be different. Japanese American men may commit suicide to avoid being a burden on their families, whereas Caucasian American men may commit suicide because of a lowered sense of self-worth resulting from retirement, or because of social isolation as a result of widowerhood and loss of work-related social networks. Diminishing health and alcohol abuse may also be contributory. Elderly women, especially African American women, appear to have strong social bonds and low rates of suicide.

Dementia

Rates of Alzheimer's dementia vary among ethnicities. For example, on the United States mainland, Alzheimer's dementia is much more common than vascular dementia. Among the Japanese American population in Hawaii, vascular dementia and Alzheimer's dementia are identical in prevalence (White et al. 1996). The incidence of risk factors for dementia may vary in different countries as a result of lifestyle rather than genetic-ethnic differences. However, genotype-phenotype relationships differ among ethnic groups, such as the relationship between apolipoprotein E type 4 allele and risk for late-onset Alzheimer's disease in whites but not in African Americans, Hispanics, or Nigerians (Tang et al. 1998).

Culturally Competent Assessment, Diagnosis, and Treatment

Clinical Assessment and Culturally Appropriate Tests

Evaluation for dementia can be difficult among ethnic-minority elderly persons with limited education. Language barriers further diminish the validity of typical tests used to evaluate whether the patient has dementia. For example, the phrase "no ifs, ands, or buts" used to test for repetition has no meaning for someone who does not speak English. Even in the multiethnic society of Hawaii, where English is the official language, such a phrase has little utility in discriminating for dementia. The substitution of a similar phrase in the patient's own language can be useful. Existing tests may have cultural biases that can adversely affect diagnosis and care. Ethnic-minority elderly persons were not among subjects used to develop diagnostic tests, and normative data for ethnic elders are often lacking (Lowenstein et al. 1994). Appropriate translation as well as determination of reliability and validity are essential. Tests such as the Cognitive Abilities Screening Instrument (Teng et al. 1994), translated versions of the Mini-Mental State Examination (Folstein et al. 1975), and the Center for Epidemiologic Studies Depression Scale (Radloff 1977) have been developed to address some of these issues.

Issues in the Care and Treatment of Elderly Patients

Psychotherapy

Psychotherapy in the elderly is quite different from psychotherapy in the younger generation (Baker and Takeshita 2001). The patient typically does not come on his or her own initiative but rather is brought by the family. The types of presenting problems are much more heterogeneous. A recent immigrant elderly individual normally has different problems than a fifth-generation elderly person of the same ethnic background. For an immigrant, English may be a second or even a third language. The formal educational background can vary from a few years to many advanced degrees.

Despite the differences among patients, there are some universal psychological themes in aging, including conflicts with adult children (the "generation gap") and declining health. Practical suggestions emphasizing here-and-now issues are particularly useful in the beginning of therapy. Discussion of somatic symptoms can serve as a venue for more psychological themes.

Transference and countertransference issues are particularly salient with the elderly. The therapist is usually younger and might even be as young as the patient's grandchildren. The patient may view the clinician as a child. On the other hand, the clinician, especially a physician, may be viewed with respect as an authority figure. Differences in age, gender, social class, and income all affect the hierarchical relationship. Countertransference issues, when the patient has parental qualities, are particularly problematic for a therapist of the same ethnicity as the patient.

Family Therapy

Working with the family is important and useful because it serves as a way to treat the patient in a natural setting. Family structure is universally present in all cultures and is a gauge of acceptable behavior, deviant behavior, and views of mental illness. It is important to determine the roles of women and men within a culture. For example, in a family meeting, it would be disastrous to assume that the elderly man is the head of the family when in fact the grandmother has that role.

Changing relationships with adult children within the life cycle is an age-old issue. As mentioned above, there tends to be a generation gap within all cultures. Elderly immigrant parents with young, acculturated children may have begun relying on the children at an early age, and this can increase the chasm. The child may function as the translator for the family, and the lack of language skills serves to further isolate the parents. Even elderly persons who have lived in the United States for decades might still understand little English, especially if contacts outside the culture have been limited.

Traditional Medicine

The use of nonallopathic medicines is common and widespread. It is now a multibillion-dollar industry and includes both traditional medicines used by people of certain cultures (e.g., kava in Polynesia) and uses by individuals outside those cultures. Regardless of one's views about nonallopathic medicines, it is important to ask about these medications because of their frequent use. Pharmacodynamic and pharmacokinetic issues are critical in the elderly and can result in toxicity, whereas the same drug did not pose a problem earlier. Traditional or nonallopathic medicine may not be viewed as a medicine per se, and it is important to specifically address this issue during the interview process.

Pharmacotherapy

Many ethnic-minority elderly persons expect to receive medications with a physician visit. For example, in Japan polypharmacy is the norm, and physicians are encouraged to prescribe medications. Unfortunately, even in the United States polypharmacy is a serious problem, and it takes quite a bit of time to educate a patient that more is not better. Injectable medications and drugs with obvious side effects may be preferred by members of certain ethnic groups because pain and discomfort are considered to be indications that the medication is powerful (Ahmed 2001).

Case Vignettes and Discussion

Case 1: An Elderly Mother Caring for a Seriously Mentally Ill Son

Mr. Randall, a 40-year-old Japanese-Caucasian man, presented to a psychiatric clinic for evaluation of psychosis. His 70-year-old widowed Japanese mother accompanied him. Mr. Randall had been slow in school in Japan and had required special education classes. His other siblings were successful attorneys. His Caucasian father had passed away many years previously. He lived with his mother, who functioned as his caretaker. Both his mother and the patient spoke primarily Japanese. Evaluation by a Japanese-speaking psychiatrist revealed a young man who had had marked auditory hallucinations for nearly 20 years but had never been treated. He was socially isolated, with no friends, although negative symptoms of schizophrenia were not prominent. He spent all of his time with his mother. Mr. Randall was referred to a Japanese-speaking psychologist for supportive therapy, primarily to assist in psychosocial rehabilitation. The mother insisted on attending all sessions with the psychologist and psychiatrist, continuing to treat her grown son as if he were a child and answering questions that were posed to the patient. Mr. Randall and his mother acknowledged significant improvement when asked in Japanese. The mother always bowed during the evaluation and expressed gratitude for being seen and receiving medications. However, to a physician who spoke only English, the patient described voices that were still prominent and that sometimes bothered him even more than before.

In this vignette, the elderly mother is the caregiver of a seriously mentally ill son. Perhaps due to the stigma of mental illness and inability to speak English, she did not seek treatment for her son for years. By the time the patient was brought in for treatment, he was floridly psychotic. Most families would have brought a family member for treatment much earlier. Although the patient was legally an adult, the elderly mother continued to treat the son as if he were a small child, possibly due to his mental illness. The filial duties were reversed here, with the young man being cared for by the elderly parent. Although the Japanese-speaking physician was young, the mother viewed him as an authority figure. As a result, she did not complain of the worsening symptoms of psychosis and continued to express gratitude for treatment. The son, on the other hand, despite his illness, became gradually acculturated, spoke some English, and, when given the opportunity, freely reported his symptoms.

Case 2: Conflict in Expectations of Care for the Elderly

Mr. Chu, a previously healthy 85-year-old, widowed Chinese man, was admitted to the hospital with a frontal lobe stroke. Evaluation revealed minimal motor problems but significant problems with executive functioning, as evidenced by poor planning and personality change. He was now quite belligerent, whereas previously he had always been pleasant. At the time of discharge from the hospital, he clearly required constant supervision. His only son wanted Mr. Chu to live with him. The son expected his stay-at-home, Caucasian wife to take care of his father. However, his wife wanted her father-in-law to be placed in a nursing facility rather than living with them. She emphasized that she would do the same even with her own parents.

This case illustrates a conflict due to cultural differences in the expectations of care for the elderly. In a traditional Asian culture, the elderly continue to live in the home environment. The emphasis on the extended family in an Asian society makes such an arrangement more acceptable. On the other hand, in Western societies, the use of nursing homes and hired help tends to be more typical. The nuclear family structure often does not allow for sufficient family members to be a in a caregiving role. The cost of long-term care in Western countries, including the United States, has reached a crisis stage. Some families reluctantly pursue family care, not because of cultural concerns, but due to finances. In Japan, nursing homes are rapidly being built as the population ages and the traditional structure of caring for the elderly is no longer practical. There is, of course, significant emotional and societal stress when finances dictate such a choice.

Case 3: Cultural Misunderstandings in a Medical Setting

Mr. Weinstein, a 72-year-old American Jewish businessman in Hawaii, was referred for depression and suicidal ideation. The surgical resident, who had been born and raised in Hawaii, noted rapid speech. Convinced that the patient had mania, the resident wanted the psychiatric consultant to administer lithium. Mr. Weinstein reported a long history of depressed moods in the context of worsening medical illness (heart failure, infections, and multiple failed surgeries). He had never taken any psychiatric medications. His wife was a Korean woman whom he had met while stationed in Korea in the military. The nursing staff reported frequent arguments between Mr. Weinstein and his wife. There were also allegations of physical assault by both husband and wife. In interviews, Mr. Weinstein's speech was rapid but not pressured. He said he was from New York City and that everyone there speaks fast. He frequently complained to the nursing staff about leg pain and stated that he was going to call Dr. Kevorkian for assistance. He emphasized that he was not suicidal and that he was just kidding. The predominantly Filipino nursing staff complained that Mr. Weinstein was rude and demanding. However, rather than confronting the patient and setting limits, they gave in to his many requests. Efforts by a Caucasian clinical nurse specialist to help the nursing staff were not successful. Mr. Weinstein's depression improved somewhat with antidepressants and better pain control, but he continued to make provocative comments and unreasonable demands.

This vignette illustrates the complexity of conflicts with multiple cultures. A regional difference in speech is misinterpreted as a sign of mania instead of a normal variant. Within this Korean-Jewish marriage, conflicts have been constant and have been handled in an aggressive and now possibly assaultive manner. Such a style works poorly with the Filipino nursing staff, who do not want to set firm limits. The result was that the patient complained and joked loudly most of the time, and the nurses were frustrated with his behavior.

Case 4: Informing a Patient of a Cancer Diagnosis

Mrs. Saito, a 75-year-old Japanese national, was visiting her daughter in the United States when she became ill. She was admitted to the hospital with complications from cancer. A psychiatrist was consulted because the daughter asked that her mother not be told that she had cancer. Mrs. Saito had previously received all her medical care in Japan. Members of the nursing staff felt that the patient had a right to know about the diagnosis and were uncomfortable with not discussing it openly. The ethics committee had concerns about informed consent. The daughter insisted that in Japan the diagnosis of cancer is not openly discussed and communicated to the patient. The psychiatrist held a family meeting with Mrs. Saito, her daughter, and the relevant staff members. Mrs. Saito acknowledged knowing about the cancer diagnosis, even in Japan. She stated that she did not tell her daughter that she knew in order to protect her daughter from worrying about her.

In Japan, the diagnosis of cancer still carries a stigma and a taboo, similar to the social environment of the 1950s and 1960s in the United States. Although this is slowly changing, the ideas of informed consent and patients' rights are still mainly American concepts, although relatively new ones. In Japan the patient frequently knows about the diagnosis of cancer, although it may not be explicitly discussed. Much is understood without direct communication.

Case 5: Intergenerational Issues Relating to Acculturation

Mr. Kumar, a 75-year-old Hindu man from India, had immigrated in his 20s to the West Coast of the United States to further his education and start a new life. After finishing graduate school he married a Caucasian Catholic woman, and the couple raised their children as Catholics. Mr. Kumar had a long and distinguished career as an academic scientist. His wife died after 45 years of marriage, and he became depressed. His grown children did their best to help him through his grief, but they felt overwhelmed as his health failed and he became more dependent on them. The oldest son and his new American wife moved in with Mr. Kumar. The couple wanted to start a family and a new life together, but Mr. Kumar said that it was the oldest son's responsibility to take care of him. This was part of their Indian heritage. Mr. Kumar's children were surprised, as they had assumed that their father was quite Westernized. They did not realize that he would revert to his Indian beliefs as he got older and sicker. They acknowledged that their father espoused Western values of independence and self-reliance; however, he had raised them in an authoritarian fashion and expected them to obey him. He used to tell them that he had been raised that way. Speaking back to him was considered disrespectful. The children felt that their father needed to be placed in a nursing home, but they were afraid to broach the subject with him. They felt intimidated and did not want their father to think they were failing in their duties as children (particularly the older son). They wondered if the doctor would tell their father that he had to be placed in a nursing home for medical reasons, but they did not want this to be presented as their wish. The psychiatrist had a joint meeting with the patient and his children, where he took the lead in raising the issue of nursing home placement. The patient expressed disappointment in his situation but was able to hear from his children that they planned to visit him regularly and remain involved in his life.

This case illustrates cultural identity, acculturation issues associated with transcultural migration, and intergenerational conflict around expectations and reality in the care of an elderly parent.

Suggestions for Clinical Practice

1. *Look at the patient as an individual.* It is very easy to stereotype on the basis of ethnicity or assumptions regarding extent of acculturation. Evaluate specific life experiences as part of the cultural assessment.
2. *Do not assume cultural explanations for behavior.* Suspiciousness, for example, may represent the emergence of paranoid delusions rather than a cultural influence. Increasing rates of dementia are common in all cultures.
3. *Involve family members in the treatment.* Family members support the patient and provide a specific framework for behaviors that are considered normal or aberrant. For the ethnic-minority elderly patient, the offspring may assume particularly defined roles, such as caregiver, spokesperson, or decision maker. These roles may rest in the same child or may be assumed by different children.
4. *Explore intergenerational issues.* The generation gap or conflict is universal but is especially an issue with immigrant ethnic-minority elderly persons, whose children may not share traditional values.
5. *Look at acculturation issues.* The amount of time in a host country is not always an indication of acculturation. Values from the home country typically affect views about mental illness.

6. *Obtain a cultural history,* including details regarding age at immigration, reasons for immigration, and background in the host country, such as rural versus urban, social status, continuing family contacts in the home country, and integration into the host country. Determine the onset of psychopathology, which may predate the immigration process.
7. *Find out about cohort experiences.* An understanding of immigration laws, prejudice, and discrimination is important in understanding a patient's cultural background.
8. *Evaluate cultural identity issues.* The cultural identification may not be synonymous with the ethnic background of the individual.
9. *Interpret cognitive tests carefully* because of potentially decreased reliability and validity. If possible, use culturally validated scales. If these are not available, one may need to improvise with culturally acceptable tests of cognition.
10. *Explore definitions of illness,* cultural expressions of illness, and expectations of the treatment relationship. Elaboration of somatic complaints may offer a good way to assess for psychiatric illness.
11. *Be clear about what is expected.* The elderly person may expect to be given a pill or injection and may be confused with the "talking cure" or individual psychotherapy. The use of alternative treatments or traditional medicine should be closely monitored for adverse effects or drug interactions.
12. *Be alert to cultural transference/countertransference issues,* especially when the patient and clinician share the same background. Issues such as overidentification can be significant.
13. *Be aware of barriers to use of services.* Social service organizations are often poorly utilized by minority elders, who may have difficulty with access or may be embarrassed to receive help. Culturally based organizations can be particularly helpful. The idea of institutionalized care can conflict with cultural expectations of home-based care.

References

Ahmed I: Aging and psychopathology, in Culture and Psychopathology: A Guide to Clinical Assessment. Edited by Tseng WS, Streltzer J. New York, Brunner/Mazel, 1997, pp 221–239

Ahmed I: Psychological aspects of giving and receiving medications, in Culture and Psychotherapy: A Guide to Clinical Practice. Edited by Tseng WS, Streltzer J. Washington, DC, American Psychiatric Press, 2001, pp 123–134

American Psychiatric Association: Diagnostic and Statistical Manual of Mental Disorders, 4th Edition, Text Revision. Washington, DC, American Psychiatric Association, 2000

Baker FM: Suicide among ethnic minority elderly: a statistical and psychosocial perspective. J Geriatr Psychiatry 27:241–264, 1994

Baker FM, Lightfoot OB: Psychiatric care of the elderly, in Culture, Ethnicity, and Mental Illness. Edited by Gaw AC. Washington, DC, American Psychiatric Press, 1993, pp 517–552

Baker FM, Takeshita J: Psychotherapy with the elderly, in Culture and Psychotherapy: A Guide to Clinical Practice. Edited by Tseng WS, Streltzer J. Washington, DC, American Psychiatric Press, 2001, pp 209–221

Braun KL, Pietsch JH, Blanchette PL (eds): Cultural Issues in End-of-Life Decision Making. Thousand Oaks, CA, Sage, 2000

Chiarolanza CCP: Attempting elder care for Japan's senior population. Long Term Care Interface, April 2001, pp 34–38

Folstein MF, Folstein ST, McHugh PR: "Mini-Mental State": a practical method for grading the cognitive stage of patients for the clinician. J Psychiatr Res 12:189–198, 1975

Freed AO: Discussion: minority elderly. J Geriatr Psychiatry 25:105–111, 1992

Fry CL: Theories of age and culture, in Emerging Theories of Aging. Edited by Birren JE, Bengston VL. Berlin, Springer-Verlag, 1988, pp 447–481

Gelfand DE: Aging and Ethnicity: Knowledge and Services. New York, Springer, 1994

Guttman D: Parenthood: a key to the comparative study of the life cycle, in Life-Span Developmental Psychology: Normative Life Crises. Edited by Datan N, Ginsberg LH. New York, Academic Press, 1975, pp 167–184

Lowenstein DA, Arguelles T, Arguelles S, et al: Potential cultural bias in neuropsychological assessment of the older adult. J Clin Exp Neuropsychol 16:623–629, 1994

Markides KS, Liang J, Jackson JS: Race, ethnicity, and aging: conceptual and methodological issues, in Handbook of Aging and the Social Sciences. Edited by Binstock RH, George LK. San Diego, CA, Academic Press, 1990, pp 112–125

Radloff LS: The CES-D scale: a self-report depression scale for research in the general population. Applied Psychological Measurement 1:383–401, 1977

Sakauye K: Ethnocultural aspects, in Comprehensive Review of Geriatric Psychiatry, 2nd Edition. Edited by Sadavoy J, Lazarus LW, Jarvik LF, et al. Washington, DC, American Psychiatric Press, 1996, pp 197–221

Tang MX, Stern Y, Marder K, et al: The APOE-epsilon 4 allele and the risk of Alzheimer disease among African Americans, whites, and Hispanics. JAMA 279:751–755, 1998

Teng EL, Hasegawa K, Homma A, et al: The Cognitive Abilities Screening Instrument (CASI): a practical test for cross-cultural epidemiological studies of dementia. Int Psychogeriatr 6:45–58, 1994

Thomas D: The Poems of Dylan Thomas. New York, New Directions, 1952

U.S. Administration on Aging: Facts and Figures: Statistics on Minority Aging in the U.S. Washington, DC, U.S. Department of Health and Human Services, 2003. Available at: http://www.aoa.gov/prof/Statistics/minority_aging/facts_minority_aging.asp. Accessed February 1, 2004.

White L, Petrovich H, Ross GW, et al: Prevalence of dementia in older Japanese-American men in Hawaii: the Honolulu-Asia Aging Study. JAMA 276:955–960, 1996

Zisook S, Shuchter SR: Grief and bereavement, in Comprehensive Review of Geriatric Psychiatry, 2nd Edition. Edited by Sadavoy J, Lazarus LW, Jarvik LF, et al. Washington, DC, American Psychiatric Press, 1996, pp 529–565

10

Culture and Drug Therapy

Keh-Ming Lin, M.D., M.P.H.
Todd S. Elwyn, M.D., J.D.

Introduction: Historical Trends

The advent of chlorpromazine and other psychotropic agents ushered psychiatry into a new era. Prescribing and managing medications has become an increasingly important part of the clinician's work, necessitating the development of expertise in the use and dosing of these new drugs. Cultural and ethnic differences that can significantly affect the effectiveness of pharmacotherapy deserve careful consideration (Lin et al. 1993).

The history of cross-ethnic and cross-cultural psychopharmacology began with some early observations by astute clinicians treating non-Caucasian populations that patients of different races or ethnicities responded differently to medications (Kalow 1989; Murphy 1969). The case reports and anecdotal observations, although they were initially treated with skepticism (Lin 1996), eventually gave way to more rigorous scientific testing. Biological factors, both genetic and nongenetic, influencing response to medication and development of side effects have been extensively researched. Over the past dozen years researchers have developed a robust understanding of the role played by these factors in producing differences in response between persons of differing ethnicity (Lin and Poland 1995; Lin and Smith 2000; Lin et al. 1995, 2001).

Psychological, social, and cultural forces are no less important in determining the clinical outcome of prescribing psychotropic medications. Unfortunately, the understanding of cultural differences in this area is not yet so advanced. The reports in the literature do provide some guidance, however, about important cultural and psychological aspects to consider when prescribing psychotropic medication. Clinicians must be well versed in understanding both the biological and cultural factors that may enhance or diminish the effectiveness of a prescribed medication. In this chapter we review some of the factors the prescribing clinician should keep in mind with patients of various ethnic, racial, and cultural backgrounds in deciding whether or not to prescribe, in selecting the right medication, in administering the correct dose, and in monitoring for side effects and compliance.

General Cultural Factors Relating to Medication

Clinicians and patients operate within the larger cultural context that shapes their attitudes, beliefs, and expectations. A clinician and patient of the same ethnicity or culture may experience difficulties due to miscommunication or a divergence of expectations, and this possibility is further increased when the parties come from different backgrounds. The roles assumed by doctor and patient, including characteristic patterns of behavior, may vary considerably between cultures.

In many Western cultures, physicians expect the patient to have some degree of medical knowledge or sophistication. Physicians may view patients as autonomous decision makers and expect them to be able to participate in decisions about medical treatment. Physicians may assume patients will stay with one doctor throughout the course of treatment and will keep the doctor apprised of side effects or other untoward events that may occur during treatment (Tseng 2003). Patients in other cultures with less medical sophistication may violate these unwritten rules. They may change doctors or see several concurrently or sequentially, take medications sporadically, and combine Western medicines with traditional ones. They may hold different ideas about how quickly the medication is supposed to work, what kinds of side effects are acceptable, and how often to follow up. The patient's family may play a significant role in making medical decisions and ensuring the patient follows up appropriately. The culturally competent clinician must be aware that cultural forces can shape every phase of the medication management process, from the initial prescribing to long-term compliance. As a consequence, the clinician must be prepared to devote adequate time and attention to addressing these issues.

Prescribing Psychotropic Medications

Deciding to Prescribe Medication

The degree of involvement by patients in medical decision making varies across cultures. In the United States, legal and ethical principles of informed consent dictate that patients must be informed of the various medical options and be empowered to choose the ones they prefer. Physicians in other countries may use a less collaborative approach such that patients come to expect the physician to make important decisions regarding prescribing. Attempts to involve such patients in the decision-making process may be less welcome and may be regarded as shifting the physician's burden onto a patient who is ill-equipped to handle it. Moreover, family members may object to the physician's fully disclosing to the patient the nature and treatment of his or her illness without consulting them first. Some diagnoses, such as schizophrenia or other chronic mental illnesses, may carry such stigma that family members would prefer that they be told but the patient be spared the devastating news. The clinician must carefully negotiate the requirements of informed consent under the local jurisdiction with the cultural expectations of the patient and family. An example of this kind of situation is presented later in this section (see "Case 1: Fear of Medication for Schizophrenia").

The act of providing medication to a patient may carry with it important symbolic meanings. For the physician, prescribing may be the concrete manifestation of the physician's power to heal the sick. The physician may also resort to medication when there is no other easy way to help the patient or when the physician is unsure of what to do (Tseng 2003). For the patient, receiving medication may demonstrate that the physician is concerned about or cares for the patient. In most cultures, medications themselves have certain powers or potencies that are transferred to the patient who takes them (Ahmed 2001). On the other hand, among groups who see doctors as "pill pushers," an overly aggressive approach to medication may undermine the therapeutic alliance.

Case 1: Fear of Medication for Schizophrenia

Mrs. Lee, a 28-year-old divorced Korean woman, was brought by her mother to the mental health clinic after referral from her primary care physician. Over the past 2 months she had become increasingly isolated in their apartment, had been accusing classmates of plotting against her, and had expressed the belief that the government was spying on her and trying to control her mind through a special satellite. In the mental health clinic, laboratory evaluation, including a urine drug screen, had negative results. On interview, Mrs. Lee was guarded and suspicious. She was noted to have psychotic symptoms of thought broadcasting, ideas of reference, and paranoid delusions. At this point Mrs. Lee's mother requested to speak with the psychiatrist alone. The patient gave her consent and the mother asked to be fully informed about her daughter's diagnosis, prognosis, and treatment options. On hearing of the probable diagnosis of schizophrenia, the mother asked that all information about the diagnosis be withheld from the patient.

The psychiatrist decided to tell Mrs. Lee that the medication was to help her sleep, and he reviewed with the patient and her mother the important side effects. Mrs. Lee agreed to take the antipsychotic, and her functioning improved enough that she was able to return to school. Several months later, while surfing the Internet, Mrs. Lee learned that her medication was used in treating schizophrenia. She refused to continue taking the medication, explaining that she did not think she had schizophrenia. The mother immediately brought her daughter back to the clinic. The psychiatrist agreed with Mrs. Lee that she might not have schizophrenia. He noted that the medicine she was taking could be helpful for various conditions besides schizophrenia and that it was useful in helping patients to think clearly. He suggested that because Mrs. Lee had been doing well while taking the medication she should consider continuing to take it for now. With her mother's encouragement, Mrs. Lee agreed to continue the medication.

Selecting a Proper Medication

Diagnosis

Selecting the wrong medication can lead to diminished efficacy and poor compliance. Choice of an appropriate medication must begin with a clear picture of the disease or illness being treated. Making an accurate diagnosis can be complicated by several factors, including cultural or ethnic differences. Research has shown that certain populations in the United States are more likely to receive an incorrect diagnosis. For example, African American patients in the United States are more likely to be misdiagnosed with schizophrenia and less likely to be diagnosed with an anxiety disorder than are Caucasian patients (Lawson 1996; Littlewood 1992). Similar problems of misdiagnosis may exist with regard to other ethnic minority groups, including Hispanic Americans and Asian Americans. Physicians may misinterpret symptoms found in patients who belong to ethnic groups other than their own (Lopez 1989), and there may also be ethnic differences in help-seeking behavior that contribute to such misdiagnoses.

Newer Versus Older Medications

For most psychiatric conditions, the prescribing physician may choose from a wide variety of similarly efficacious treatments. Newer medications may have superior side-effect profiles to those of older medications but may cost substantially more. Although the standard of medical care and relevant clinical considerations should determine which treatment is selected, some data suggest that physicians are more likely to prescribe older medications for patients who are members of ethnic minoritygroups. For example, studies in the United States have suggested that non-Caucasian schizophrenic patients may be more likely to receive conventional antipsychotics than the newer atypical antipsychotics (Kuno and Rothbard 2002; Owen et al. 2001; Valenstein et al. 2001). In one study, depressed African American patients were more likely than Caucasian patients to be prescribed older tricyclic antidepressants rather than the newer selective serotonin reuptake inhibitors (Melfi et al. 2000). However, not all studies have revealed statistically significant differences in prescribing patterns by ethnicity for schizophrenic patients (Woods et al. 2003) or for depressed outpatients (Sleath et al. 2001).

Religious Considerations

People may observe certain rules, customs, or taboos in their daily lives or may hold certain views that are rooted in their religious or secular beliefs. Religious proscriptions applied to how medications are prepared may limit the choice of medications that may be used. For example, Muslims may not use medications containing alcohol. Muslims and orthodox Jews object to taking medications in which porcine products were used (Ahmed 2001). Strict vegetarians or vegans may be unwilling to take any medications containing animal products.

Placebo Effects

Physical characteristics of the medication itself—such as its color, size, route of administration, and taste—may (unexpectedly to the physician) alter the strength of the placebo effect of the medication on the patient. For example, one study found that African American subjects were more likely to view black capsules as analgesics and white capsules as stimulants. Conversely, Caucasians were more likely to regard black capsules as stimulants and white ones as analgesics (Buckalew and Caulfield 1982). Asian patients and those from developing countries may believe that injectable medications are the most potent and therefore expect and prefer them to orally administered medicines (Kleinman 1980; Reeler 1990). In some countries medication is often in the form of a powder, and the patient may expect that one or more powders will be used (Nunley 1996).

Medication Dosage: Psychopharmacological Perspectives

Dosing of medications is affected by a variety of factors, both biological and nonbiological. The biological factors can be divided into genetic and nongenetic factors. Biological factors such as pharmacokinetics and pharmacodynamics are affected by race or ethnicity.

Pharmacokinetics and Pharmacodynamics

Pharmacodynamics and pharmacokinetics determine the effects of psychotropic agents and account for differences in response between individuals (interindividual variation) and between races or ethnicities (cross-ethnic or cross-racial variations). *Pharmacodynamics* refers to the drugs' effects on receptors in the body to produce a pharmacological effect. *Pharmacokinetics* refers to how the body handles the drug with regard to absorption, distribution, metabolism, and excretion. Of these factors, variation in metabolism is thought to account for most of the variation in response (Lin et al. 2001).

Genetic Factors

Metabolism of most psychotropic agents proceeds through the cytochrome P450 system. The cytochrome P450 enzymes most commonly involved are CYP1A2, CYP2C19, CYP2D6, and CYP3A4. Because of genetic polymorphism (i.e., different forms of the same enzyme) the activity of cytochrome P450 enzymes varies considerably between individuals and across populations. This genetic heterogeneity, which is assumed to be evolutionarily adaptive for a population in meeting diverse environmental challenges, accounts for much of the difference in pharmacological effect (Lin et al. 1995; Smith and Mendoza 1996).

Individuals can be classified on the basis of genetic polymorphism into one of four categories: poor metabolizers, who are unable to produce the cytochrome P450 enzyme; intermediate metabolizers, who have only one fully functioning allele or who possess variant alleles with less enzyme activity; extensive metabolizers, who possess two normally functioning alleles; and ultrarapid metabolizers, who have three or more fully functioning alleles (Lin et al. 2001). Poor metabolizers may have increased drug plasma concentrations as a result of impaired metabolism and therefore require a lower dose to avoid unwanted side effects. Conversely, ultrarapid metabolizers will metabolize the drug rapidly and require a higher dose to avoid therapeutic failure.

Clinically significant genetic polymorphisms have been found for every enzyme studied. The distribution of these various cytochrome P450 alleles has been shown to vary considerably across race and ethnicity. Perhaps the best-studied of these is the CYP2D6 enzyme. More than 50 alleles for CYP2D6 with functional significance have been found. The *CYP2D6*4* allele is found mostly in Caucasians with European ancestry and is responsible for poor drug metabolism in 5%–9% of this population. The *CYP2D6*10* allele, which also results in impaired functioning, is found in as many as 70% of East Asians, but it is not common in other groups. In persons of African heritage, the allele *CYP2D6*17* is associated with reduced enzymatic activity. These alleles are thought to account for the lower therapeutic dose ranges for tricyclic antidepressants in African Americans and Asians and for the lower dose range for antipsychotics in Asians (Lin and Poland 1995; Lin et al. 1988). The prevalence of CYP2D6 ultrarapid metabolism also varies by ethnicity. Among Arabs and Ethiopians, the prevalence is 20%–30%, far more than the 1%–5% among Europeans.

The other common cytochrome P450 enzymes show similar heterogeneity. The benzodiazepine diazepam and the antidepressant citalopram are metabolized by CYP2C19. Because of differences in alleles, 20% of East Asians but only 3%–5% of Caucasians are poor metabolizers (Goldstein et al. 1997; Lin et al. 2001). Ethnic differences in the activity of CYP1A2 and CYP3A4 enzymes have also been discovered. A final point to note is that ethnic variability in genes affecting therapeutic targets of psychotropic medications, such as the serotonin transporter and the serotonin or dopamine receptors, may account for differential responses to treatment.

Case 2: A Patient Who Is an Ultrarapid Metabolizer

Miss Eshete, a 20-year-old Ethiopian woman with paranoid schizophrenia, chronic type, moved to the United States after beginning treatment with chlorpromazine in Ethiopia. Her medication was changed to risperidone to address her persistent paranoid ideation, and the dose was gradually increased from 0.5 mg twice a day to 4 mg at night over the course of 3 months. With a risperidone dose of 4 mg/day the patient had not improved, and plasma levels of risperidone and its metabolite 9-hydroxy-risperidone were measured. No detectable plasma levels of the parent compound were noted, and 17 ng/mL of the metabolite was detected. The dose of risperidone was gradually increased to 12 mg/ day with no improvement in positive or negative symptoms and no increase in plasma levels over those found at the 4-mg/day dose. At that time, a known CYP2D6 inhibitor, paroxetine (10 mg/day), was added to the medication regimen. When the paroxetine ws started, the risperidone dose was increased to 16 mg/day, and within 3 days the patient's positive and negative symptoms improved. She was able to obtain employment, but she had pronounced positive symptoms at night. At a risperidone dose of 16 mg/day (plus paroxetine) the patient developed symptomatic orthostatic hypotension and lost her job. The risperidone dose was eventually adjusted to 12 mg/day and the paroxetine dose to 20 mg twice a day. At these doses the patient had no positive or negative symptoms and did not exhibit any extrapyramidal symptoms for 7 months. The plasma level of the parent compound was measured as 3.3 ng/mL, and the metabolite concentration was 40 ng/mL. A genotyping test revealed that the patient was an ultrarapid metabolizer of drugs metabolized by CYP2D6 because she possessed more than two copies of the gene (gene duplication). (Case contributed by M. Smith and L. Workneh, personal communication, August 2003.)

As noted earlier, the prevalence of ultrarapid metabolism is exceptionally high (29%) among Ethiopians. This case suggests that close to one-third of North Africans and Middle Easterners might encounter similar problems when treated with medications that depend on CYP2D6 for their metabolism.

Nongenetic Biological Factors

A number of nongenetic biological factors, such as age or sex, have been shown to affect the metabolism of medications. For example, aging is often associated with a significant decline in the activity of some of the cytochrome P450 enzymes, resulting in higher plasma levels of medications (Salzman 1984). Other factors related to culture or ethnicity—such as diet, smoking, and the use of herbal compounds—have also been shown to have pharmacological effects. Just as medications can inhibit or induce cytochrome P450 enzymes to produce drug interactions, foods and other substances are also metabolized through the cytochrome P450 system and can affect the metabolism of prescribed medications. Contemporaneous consumption of such compounds and prescribed medications may result in either overdosing and the development of side effects or underdosing and therapeutic failure.

Activity of the CYP1A2 enzyme can be induced by a high-protein diet and inhibited by a diet high in carbohydrates (Branch et al. 1978). Other compounds inducing CYP1A2 include cruciferous vegetables such as cabbage and sprouts, those with aromatic hydrocarbons such as charbroiled beef, and smoking tobacco. The effect of diet on the response to medication was seen in Asian Indian subjects consuming a vegetarian diet. When they changed to a British diet, their pharmacokinetic profiles for some medications changed to resemble those of the British (Allen et al. 1977).

The CYP3A4 enzyme has been shown to be inhibited by a variety of natural substances, including grapefruit juice and other substances containing bioflavonoids. At the same time, other natural substances exert a strong inducing effect on this enzyme. This is best exemplified in the case of *Hypericum* (St. John's wort), an herbal preparation that has been widely used for the treatment of mild depression. When used in combination with other drugs that are metabolized by CYP3A4, St. John's wort has been found to significantly reduce the blood levels of these drugs. These examples indicate that in addition to their pharmacological properties, many herbal medicines could also modulate the pharmacokinetics and pharmacodynamics of prescribed medications, leading to unexpected toxicity or loss of efficacy.

Case 3: A Patient With Dementia From Herbal Medicine

Mrs. Rizal, a 75-year-old Filipino American woman, was referred to a geriatric psychiatrist for cognitive deficits. Evaluation revealed significant memory deficits and other features consistent with a dementia. The psychiatrist took a thorough inventory of medications and supplements, and Mrs. Rizal admitted taking an herbal tea for many years, believing that it was an herbal medicine that was good for her health. The ingredients of this tea had significant anticholinergic effects, however, that caused her to develop cognitive problems. Her cognition dramatically improved after discontinuing the herbal medicine.

This vignette illustrates the importance of taking a thorough inventory of all substances being used—including modern, traditional, and folk medicines. Traditional medicines, both those prescribed by healers and those purchased over the counter, have significant pharmacological effects. By themselves, they can have serious side effects. In combination with prescribed medications, the drug interaction profile can become toxic.

Nonbiological Factors

Some have suggested that differences in the effect of medications are influenced by the personality or cultural background of the patient. People from cultures that are thought to be more competitive, emotional, and aggressive are believed to require more medication than those from cultures that are more peaceful, easygoing, and relaxed. Chinese, for example, are said to require higher doses of antipsychotic medication for schizophrenia than Malays, who are viewed as less aggressive in general in their approaches to life (Murphy 1969). This effect, on a national level, echoes the literature on expressed emotion, suggesting that patients whose families are high in expressed emotion require more antipsychotic medication (Ahmed 2001).

Side Effects

The failure to adequately take into account the biological factors affecting dosing may result in side effects at doses lower than expected. For example, Asian patients taking typical antipsychotics may develop extrapyramidal symptoms at lower doses than Caucasians (Binder and Levy 1981). One study suggested that in treating Asian patients with schizophrenia, switching to the atypical antipsychotic olanzapine can improve the side-effect profile (C. T. Lee et al. 2002). Beyond biological factors, placebo effects often play a role in the perception or reporting of side effects, with some cultures finding certain side effects more distressing than others. For example, one study found that Hong Kong Chinese patients taking lithium rarely complain about the kinds of side effects that Western patients typically dislike, including weight gain and loss of creativity. In fact, patients viewed the troublesome side effects of polydipsia and polyuria positively, as evidence that the medicine was working (S. Lee 1993). The view that traditional medications and herbal preparations are less potent but safer than Western medicines may also influence perceptions about their respective side effects.

Compliance and Follow-up

Physicians from all disciplines and in all countries struggle with the issue of noncompliance. Among non-Western populations in Western nations, where there may be communication difficulties and a disparity between beliefs of patient and physician, the problem may be even greater (Smith et al. 1993). A variety of cultural differences may affect a patient's perceptions about the need to continue taking medication. For example, in China it is widely believed that Western medicines are very powerful and work quickly to relieve symptoms. If the medications do not achieve results in two or three visits, the patient will regard them as having failed and will change doctors (Kleinman 1980). Moreover, the effect of choosing a medication that is at odds with traditional beliefs will worsen compliance. For example, a medication that makes a patient feel weak will not be well received by a patient who believes his sickness stems from a loss of vitality (Tseng 2003). Traditional folk beliefs about the causes of illness that are not rooted in modern science may result in noncompliance with prescribed medication regimens (Ahmed 2001). When medications are at odds with beliefs from traditional medical systems, for whatever reason, they are at risk of being discontinued.

The influence of family on the patient's compliance cannot be ignored. For patients from cultures that prize family interdependence, family members can help facilitate compliance by bringing the patient to scheduled appointments or by holding and dispensing medications. This may be especially important with patients who have psychosis, severe depression, or dementia and who otherwise might omit to follow up with care, forget to take medicine, or take it inappropriately. In some cases, family members may become overinvolved and even sabotage treatment (Canive et al. 2001). The perceptions, attitudes, and beliefs of family members toward taking medications prescribed by the physician will have a direct impact on the patient's compliance. In fact, the family's influence may determine whether or not the patient takes the prescribed medicine. How family members view a medication, and the interactional relations between patient and family, become important questions for clinical practice. Furthermore, educating and involving family members in the decision-making process can help establish a positive alliance with the family that will translate to improved compliance. The following case illustrates these points.

Case 4: A Patient Who Followed the Advice of His Elder Sister Rather Than the Directives of the Physician

Mr. Lopez, a 40-year-old married Hispanic American man, had received a prescription for an antidepressant from his psychiatrist for treatment of depression. At first he was very reluctant to continue taking the medication because of great concern about the side effects he developed, including dry mouth, blurred vision, and mild dyspepsia. Through his wife's support and encouragement and his psychiatrist's advice, Mr. Lopez finally agreed to take the medication regularly, and his depressive symptoms gradually improved. To prevent relapse into depression, the psychiatrist asked Mr. Lopez to continue taking the medicine. While visiting his hometown one day, Mr. Lopez met his elderly sister, who had raised him after the loss of their mother when he was a small boy. His sister held the folk view that Western medicine is too strong and will harm the body if taken too long. She encouraged him to stop taking the antidepressant. Instead, she advised him to use herbal medicine, which she said would function as a tonic to nourish the body in a harmonious way. Mr. Lopez did stop taking the Western antidepressant medicine, and within a month his depression recurred. He was brought to the clinic by his wife to see the psychiatrist again so that drug treatment could be restarted.

Schizophrenic patients who are poorly compliant often have long-acting injectable antipsychotics prescribed for them. This is one explanation given for why African American patients in the United States are more likely than other populations to be given long-acting depot medications (Kuno and Rothbard 2002; Price et al. 1985; Valenstein et al. 2001; Woods et al. 2003), reflecting the prevailing bias by professionals that noncompliance may be a larger problem in this population than in others. Problems with compliance may result from a variety of factors, including physician error. Misdiagnosis and prescribing the wrong medication, prescribing doses that are too high or too low, or failing to monitor for side effects are important causes that the culturally sensitive physician must consider. Poor compliance may result from patient-related or institutional factors, such as economic difficulties, lack of education or understanding, or difficulties in acquiring care. On a basic level, patients unfamiliar with the Western medical system who receive a prescription may not understand how or where to get it filled.

Patients may differ in their expectations of how frequently follow-up with the clinician should occur. In Japan, for example, physicians are restricted in the amount of medications they may prescribe, so patients must return to the clinic more frequently. Some clinicians in the United States will dispense medications for 1 month and make several refills available, particularly if the patient is stable. This practice may convey the message that the doctor does not wish to see the patient or does not care.

Additional Case Vignettes With Discussion

Case 5: The Doctor Prescribes, the Patient Does Not Take

Mrs. Takaki, a 63-year-old Japanese American woman, complained to her internal medicine physician of tremors and a movement disorder after encountering stress at work. This physician diagnosed major depression and prescribed extended-release venlafaxine, starting at 150 mg/day. The patient took the medication for a few days, but she experienced severe nausea and a skin rash and decided to stop taking it. Mrs. Takaki failed to inform her physician because of her discomfort in telling him that she did not follow his order.

Subsequently Mrs. Takaki consulted a psychiatrist for her anxiety associated with movement problems. The psychiatrist, whose clinical impression was that she had an adjustment disorder, treated her with brief supportive therapy, and her condition, including the unusual movements, improved. When Mrs. Takaki returned to the internist after 1 month, she did not tell him she had seen a psychiatrist or that she had stopped taking her medication. The physician assumed his treatment had helped ameliorate her symptoms and continued to prescribe the venlafaxine, while Mrs. Takaki continued secretly not taking it.

This vignette illustrates several aspects of culture and psychopharmacology. First, the physician incorrectly gave the patient a diagnosis of major depressive disorder. Second, the prescribed dose of medication exceeded the normal starting dose for all patients and was particularly problematic because the patient was a poor metabolizer of the medication. Third, the patient discontinued her medication but did not tell the physician she had done so. Finally, she consulted another physician and received treatment without letting the first physician know about it. Her passive personality style in addition to her cultural upbringing made it difficult for her to tell the physician—an authority figure—that she was not complying with his order.

Case 6: Sharing Medicine With Relatives

Mr. Kaipat, a 45-year-old Micronesian man, visited a physician for back pain. The doctor prescribed analgesic medication that relieved the pain. But Mr. Kaipat kept coming back to see the physician, asking for more medication. Mr. Kaipat used various excuses, saying that he had lost the medicine or that the dose was sometimes not strong enough to control the pain so he had to take it more frequently than prescribed. Because Mr. Kaipat kept asking for more, the physician suspected that he might be selling the pain medication. Later, the physician learned from family members that Mr. Kaipat was sharing his "good" medicine with his family and relatives when they had aches or pains. According to Mr. Kaipat's island culture, every one in the community should share things—including cash, food, or medicine—with family members, relatives, or even neighbors, in order to survive together on their tiny island. It was pointed out to Mr. Kaipat and his family that this was not allowed in the American medical system, because of medical insurance requirements, and particularly because it could be dangerous medically.

Case 7: One Patient, Three Therapists

Mr. Liu, a Chinese American man in his 40s, developed severe anxiety and depression after his boss scolded him for not working fast enough. Afraid that he might lose his job, Mr. Liu became very nervous and depressed. His wife took him to the emergency room, and he subsequently was hospitalized because of suicidal thoughts. A Caucasian psychiatrist treated Mr. Liu initially and prescribed an antidepressant for him at the usual starting dose, but the patient developed severe side effects. The psychiatrist suspected that Mr. Liu was manifesting features of hysteria, because he was reluctant to return to work despite being counseled by the psychiatrist as to the best way to cope with his encounter at work. Mr. Liu, frightened by the medication's side effects and worried that the therapist was "not understanding his problems correctly," asked to be discharged and to be seen by a Chinese psychiatrist who could speak his language.

The second psychiatrist, who spoke Mr. Liu's language, prescribed the same medication that had been prescribed by the first (Caucasian) psychiatrist. The patient was so afraid of this medication that he refused to take it. The psychiatrist then tried several kinds of antidepressants. However, Mr. Liu would use each of them for a day or so and then discontinue them because of the side effects. Mr. Liu began to feel that this psychiatrist did not know how to treat him and became frustrated. The second psychiatrist was frustrated as well, finding the patient to be hypochondriacal, noncompliant, and a chronic complainer. Dissatisfied with treatment progress, the second psychiatrist referred him to another Chinese psychiatrist who was highly regarded by the Chinese in the community.

The third psychiatrist, knowing what had happened to Mr. Liu, started the same antidepressant the two other psychiatrists had tried, but at a very low initial dose. He carefully explained to the patient the kinds of side effects he might develop as well as the nature and purpose of taking this medication, even though side effects might be expected initially. This psychiatrist persuaded Mr. Liu to take the medicine, convincing him that it was the best and only way to improve his depression. After developing a trusting relationship with the third psychiatrist, Mr. Liu followed the doctor's orders and took the medicine faithfully. With a gradual increase in the dose and the provision of supplemental supportive psychotherapy, Mr. Liu's depression eventually improved. (Revised from Carlton 2001)

This case illustrates that the prescription of medication by the therapist to the patient is a dynamic process that includes psychological issues beyond biological factors. Even though the same medication was chosen and prescribed by these three therapists, the patient reacted differently toward the therapists regarding the medication prescribed for him. The case illustrates the importance of the therapist-patient relationship and the psychological and cultural aspects of the giving and receiving of medication that interact with biological factors.

Suggestions for Clinical Practice

1. *Take time to learn about the cultures of the patients you are treating.* Financial pressures increasingly push physicians into the role of

"medication management." Learning about a patient's culture, however, takes time and may be impossible to accomplish during a 10- to 15-minute medication visit. Important issues for the clinician to review include the following: 1) How does the patient, according to his or her culture, view the meaning of taking medication? 2) What attitude does the patient hold toward taking Western medicine versus traditional or herbal medicine? 3) Does the patient have any beliefs about the effect of medicine? It is also useful to understand a patient's custom regarding compliance with prescribed medication regimens and whether there is any tendency to see multiple clinicians simultaneously and receive different medications from different doctors. This knowledge can help avoid undesirable drug interactions, including those resulting from taking Western and herbal medicines together.

2. *Be aware of the need to adjust medication dose according to ethnicity.* The dosing of psychotropic medicine to achieve the most desirable therapeutic effects with minimal ill effects, including side effects, will vary depending not only on the patient's body weight, age, sex, and physical condition, but also on his or her ethnic or racial background. Clinicians must be aware of the possibility that side effects will occur at lower doses than expected, or that therapeutic failure will occur at higher doses, and must make adjustments accordingly. When a patient is not responding as expected and there is a question of compliance or varied metabolism, serum levels of various medications and their metabolites can be measured to guide subsequent dosing decisions. Pharmacogenetic information—including determination of the variation patterns of genes relevant to drug responses and measurement of the activity of drug-metabolizing enzymes—may also be available in the near future to assist such decisions.

3. *Understand the dynamic nature of prescribing and receiving medication.* Prescribing and receiving medications is a dynamic, interactive process between the therapist and the patient that extends beyond mere psychopharmacological effects. It includes the relations and interactions between the therapist and the patient and involves issues of agreement, trust, and compliance. The prescription of medication reflects the exercising of authority—either symbolically or in reality—by the therapist over the patient, who consents to this relationship of unequal power in order to get well. The clinician's perception of this relationship, inasmuch as it is influenced by culture, may differ from the patient's perception. This must be considered when lack of compliance or follow-up becomes a problem.

4. *Comprehend the cultural implications of taking medication.* Patients may have culturally influenced views about the color, form, packaging, and other aspects of the medicine itself, including the route of administration (such as taking it by mouth versus by injection). Other views that are important to elicit include the patient's beliefs regarding the kind of medicine being prescribed, such as pain medicine or nutritional medicine, and the patient's reactions toward the side effects he or she experiences. In other words, the clinician must realize that the giving of medication by the therapist to the patient is a delicate and complicated matter that involves psychological and cultural considerations and not solely biological and pharmacological factors.

References

Ahmed I: Psychological aspects of giving and receiving medications, in Culture and Psychotherapy: A Guide to Clinical Practice. Edited by Tseng WS, Streltzer J. Washington, DC, American Psychiatric Press, 2001, pp 123–134

Allen JJ, Rack PH, Vaddadi KS: Differences in the effects of clomipramine on English and Asian volunteers: preliminary report on a pilot study. Postgrad Med J 53 (suppl 4):79–86, 1977

Binder RL, Levy R: Extrapyramidal reactions in Asians. Am J Psychiatry 138:1243–1244, 1981

Branch RA, Salih SY, Homeida M: Racial differences in drug metabolizing activities: a study with antipyrine in the Sudan. Clin Pharmacol Ther 24:283–286, 1978

Buckalew LW, Caulfield KE: Drug expectations associated with perceptual characteristics: ethnic factors. Percept Mot Skills 55:915–918, 1982

Canive JM, Castillo DT, Tuason VB: The Hispanic veteran, in Culture and Psychotherapy: A Guide to Clinical Practice. Edited by Tseng WS, Streltzer J. Washington, DC, American Psychiatric Press, 2001, pp 157–172

Carlton BS: One patient, three therapists, in Culture and Psychotherapy: A Guide to Clinical Practice. Edited by Tseng WS, Streltzer J. Washington, DC, American Psychiatric Press, 2001, pp 67–78

Goldstein JA, Ishizaki T, Chiba K, et al: Frequencies of the defective CYP2C19 alleles responsible for the mephenytoin poor metabolizer phenotype in various Oriental, Caucasian, Saudi Arabian and American black populations. Pharmacogenetics 7:59–64, 1997

Kalow W: Race and therapeutic drug response. N Engl J Med 320:588–589, 1989

Kleinman A: Patients and Healers in the Context of Culture. Berkeley, CA, University of California Press, 1980

Kuno E, Rothbard AB: Racial disparities in antipsychotic prescription patterns for patients with schizophrenia. Am J Psychiatry 159:567–572, 2002

Lawson WB: The art and science of the psychopharmacotherapy of African Americans. Mt Sinai J Med 63:301–305, 1996

Lee CT, Conde BJ, Mazlan M, et al: Switching to olanzapine from previous antipsychotics: a regional collaborative multicenter trial assessing 2 switching techniques in Asia Pacific. J Clin Psychiatry 63:569–576, 2002

Lee S: Side effects of chronic lithium therapy in Hong Kong Chinese: an ethnopsychiatric perspective. Cult Med Psychiatry 17:301–320, 1993

Lin KM: Psychopharmacology in cross-cultural psychiatry. Mt Sinai J Med 63:283–284, 1996

Lin KM, Poland RE: Ethnicity, culture, and psychopharmacology, in Psychopharmacology: The Fourth Generation of Progress. Edited by Bloom FE, Kupfer DI. New York, Raven, 1995, pp 1907–1917

Lin KM, Smith MW: Psychopharmacotherapy in the context of culture and ethnicity, in Ethnicity and Psychopharmacotherapy, American Psychiatric Press Review of Psychiatry, Vol 19. Edited by Ruiz P. Washington, DC, American Psychiatric Press, 2000, pp 1–36

Lin KM, Poland RE, Lau EK, et al: Haloperidol and prolactin concentrations in Asians and Caucasians. J Clin Psychopharmacol 8:195–201, 1988

Lin KM, Poland RE, Nakasaki G (eds): Psychopharmacology and Psychobiology of Ethnicity. Washington, DC, American Psychiatric Press, 1993

Lin KM, Poland RE, Anderson D: Psychopharmacology, ethnicity and culture. Transcultural Psychiatric Research Review 32:3–40, 1995

Lin KM, Smith MW, Ortiz V: Culture and psychopharmacology. Psychiatr Clin North Am 24:523–538, 2001

Littlewood R: Psychiatric diagnosis and racial bias: empirical and interpretative approaches. Soc Sci Med 34:141–149, 1992

Lopez SR: Patient variable biases in clinical judgment: conceptual overview and methodological considerations. Psychol Bull 106:184–203, 1989

Melfi CA, Croghan TW, Hanna MP, et al: Racial variation in antidepressant treatment in a Medicaid population. J Clin Psychiatry 61:16–21, 2000

Murphy HBM: Ethnic variations in drug responses. Transcultural Psychiatric Research Review 6:6–23, 1969

Nunley M: Why psychiatrists in India prescribe so many drugs. Cult Med Psychiatry 20:165–197, 1996

Owen RR, Feng WW, Thrush CR: Variations in prescribing practices for novel antipsychotic medications among Veterans Affairs hospitals. Psychiatr Serv 52:1523–1525, 2001

Price ND, Glazer WM, Morgenstern H: Race and the use of fluphenazine decanoate. Am J Psychiatry 142:1491–1492, 1985

Reeler AV: Injections: a fatal attraction. Soc Sci Med 31:1119–1125, 1990

Salzman C: Clinical Geriatric Psychopharmacology. New York, McGraw-Hill, 1984

Sleath BL, Rubin RH, Huston SA: Antidepressant prescribing to Hispanic and non-Hispanic white patients in primary care. Ann Pharmacother 35:419–423, 2001

Smith MW, Mendoza RP: Ethnicity and pharmacogenetics. Mt Sinai J Med 63:285–290, 1996

Smith M, Lin KM, Mendoza R: "Nonbiological" issues affecting psychopharmacotherapy: cultural considerations, in Psychopharmacology and Psychobiology of Ethnicity (Progress in Psychiatry series). Edited by Lin KM, Poland RE, Nakasaki G. Washington, DC, American Psychiatric Press, 1993, pp 37–58

Tseng WS: Clinician's Guide to Cultural Psychiatry. San Diego, CA, Academic Press, 2003

Valenstein M, Copeland LA, Owen R, et al: Adherence assessments and the use of depot antipsychotics in patients with schizophrenia. J Clin Psychiatry 62:545–551, 2001

Woods SW, Sullivan MC, Neuse EC, et al: Racial and ethnic effects on antipsychotic prescribing practices in a community mental health center. Psychiatr Serv 54:177–179, 2003

11

Culture and Psychotherapy

Wen-Shing Tseng, M.D.

Introduction: Culture and Psychotherapy

Modern psychiatrists have come to realize that cultural considerations are essential in the practice of psychiatry, particularly in the area of psychotherapy. Psychotherapy, as the art of psychological treatment, focuses primarily on psychological dimensions of behavior and problems and naturally includes the dimensions of culture. The new term *cultural competence* has become a buzzword among clinicians. Cultural competence requires the qualities of cultural awareness and sensitivity, cultural knowledge and information, culture-appropriate attitudes and empathy, and the ability and insight to provide culturally oriented, relevant, and effective care in mental health treatment (for more detail see Chapter 1, Introduction: Culture and Psychiatry). These basic qualities, required in various forms of clinical psychiatric service and treatment, are especially important in psychotherapy.

Approaches to the Study of Culture and Psychotherapy

Cultural psychiatrists have used various approaches to examine the cultural aspects of psychotherapy. Historically, following the path of medical anthropologists, cultural psychiatrists have studied various forms of psychological treatment, including indigenous and folk therapies, in comparison to modern, mainstream psychotherapy. Psychotherapy was defined broadly (Prince 1980), and shamanism, divination, and fortune telling were all included in the investigation. Through such comparisons, scholars revealed differences in their major orientations (from the supernatural, natural, or medical-somatic to the psychological), therapeutic operations (such as healing ceremonies, symbolic interpretation, instruction, obtaining new life experience, analytical interpretation, and behavior manipulation), and healing mechanisms (such as magical counteracting, emotional catharsis, suggestions, reexamination of the self, changes in attitudes and views, and attainment of insight) (Tseng 1999). However, it has been pointed out that despite these differences, certain therapeutic mechanisms are common to various modes of psychological treatment. Frank (1961) pointed out that it is within the therapist's ability to arouse hope for recovery. Torrey (1986) has indicated that whether healers are traditional or modern, they are able to decrease the client's anxiety by identifying what is wrong, naming the cause of the problems, presenting certain personal qualities that are admired by the culture, and providing the client with a sense of learning and mastery through therapy.

The impact of culture on psychotherapy has also been studied according to the vicissitudes of psychotherapies observed in various countries and societies. These examinations vividly revealed the impact of society and culture on psychotherapy as well. One of the best examples is the way psychotherapy was discouraged in Germany during the Nazi regime, with the party's stated reason that the people had no need for psychotherapy, particularly not an analytical psychotherapy invented by a Jew. In China before the Cultural Revolution, individual psychotherapy, particularly the Western psychoanalytical variety, was severely criticized and forbidden as a product of Western capitalism. Intended merely for affluent persons, it was not suitable for a group-oriented, socialistic society. The psychoanalysis invented in Vienna during the Victorian era did not become popular there because of the conservative cultural environment. It was well accepted, instead, in the New World, where the cultural emphasis was on freedom and liberal movements, with the promise of individual actualization and achievement. Such historical observations have revealed that in addition to being influenced by medical knowledge and professional experience, the practice of psychotherapy is subject to the impact of political ideology, social background, and cultural trends that prevail in a society at a given period of time.

Stimulated by the human rights movement in the 1960s, there was increased concern in the United States with providing culturally suitable and relevant psychotherapy for patients with ethnic or cultural backgrounds different from their therapists'. This was noted to be particularly important when the therapist belongs to the majority ethnic group and the patient to an ethnic minority. The cultural influence on psychotherapy was examined in detail at a microscopic level through intercultural psychotherapy, which was concerned with how cultural factors affect the process of psychotherapy. It included a patient's orientation and expectation of psychotherapy, communication between the therapist and the patient, the therapist-patient relationship, assessment and understanding of the problems presented, interpretation and advice giving, and the goal of therapy (Tseng 2001).

The Need for Culturally Competent Psychotherapy

It has become a matter of common sense that psychotherapy needs to be adjusted according to the social, ethnic, and cultural background of the patients. Providing relevant psychotherapy across cultures is a major concern for clinicians serving patients of diverse backgrounds (Pedersen et al. 1996). This is especially true when the society is composed of multiethnic groups (Tseng and Streltzer 2001). However, even in a society that claims to be a monoculture, composed of people of homogeneous backgrounds, a careful look reveals that the members of the society belong to different subcultural groups based on socioeconomic levels, educational or occupational backgrounds, or urban-rural geographical factors. Furthermore, a society is not static in terms of culture; it is always subject to cultural change, resulting in changes in views and value systems over time and between different generations. In other words, most societies are heterogeneous in terms of cultural or subcultural matters.

Following this logic, we may say that every person has his or her own individual culture, associated with individual personal background and development, as well as personal experiences of acculturation beyond the contributing factors of personality, intelligence, or personal life experiences. Thus, as pointed out by Wohl (1989), all psychotherapy is "intercultural" in that no two people have identical, internalized constructions of their cultural worlds. Cultural issues tend to be noticed only when cultural differences between the patient and the therapist are clearly evident. In reality there is no sharp difference between intracultural and intercultural psychotherapy. They are merely different locations on a continuum. Thus, all psychotherapy needs to be culturally relevant.

Technical, Theoretical, and Philosophical Considerations

It is apparent that psychotherapy should always be practiced in a way that is relevant to the patient and to the social setting where the practice takes place, including political background, social class, economic situation, ethnic and racial factors, and cultural diversity. The carrying out of culture-relevant and culture-competent psychotherapy requires adjustments on three levels: technical, theoretical, and philosophical (Tseng 1995).

Technical Adjustments

Technical adjustments in psychotherapy include the need for the therapist to make proper choices regarding skills or techniques in therapy to fit the background of the patient. They include adequate preparation for therapy, suitable adjustment of the therapist-patient relationship, careful management of ethnic and cultural transference and countertransference, culturally relevant communication and interpretation, proper selection of modes of therapy, and relevant selection of the goals of therapy. Most clinicians and scholars have focused on these technical modifications in transcultural or intercultural psychotherapy.

Theoretical Adjustments

Beyond technical adjustments, it is also necessary to make conceptual or theoretical modifications to therapy to fit the patient's cultural background. Ethnicity and culture are to be recognized as significant parameters in understanding psychological processes. At present, several theories, particularly psychoanalytical ones, are utilized by therapists to understand the patient's personality and behavior. However, these theories are subject to cross-cultural modifications if they are to be used for people living in different sociocultural settings. Some examples are concepts of self and ego boundaries, theories of personality development, theories of defense mechanisms, and therapeutic mechanisms concerning expression or suppression.

Philosophical Considerations

In the practice of intercultural psychotherapy, the therapist needs to take into consideration the patient's (as well as the therapist's) philosophical orientation. A patient's fundamental views of and attitudes toward human beings, society, and life—closely related to concepts of normality, maturity, and health—will have obvious effects on the patient in his or her search for improvement. Furthermore, the philosophical understanding of suffering and problems and culturally determined choices for the resolution of problems will shape the course and goals of therapy. In addition, the therapist's own value system and philosophical attitudes toward life and problems will explicitly or implicitly guide the direction of therapy, particularly regarding ways to encourage the patient to resolve his or her problems and to set up the goals of treatment.

Cultural Considerations in Various Modes of Psychotherapy

Cultural psychiatrists take into account cultural considerations in various modes of psychotherapy, from individual to interpersonal therapy. Through such discussions, the knowledge and experience can be easily translated into actual clinical application (Tseng 2003). Described below are some of the major modes of psychotherapy recognized in the field.

Supportive Therapy

By definition, *supportive psychotherapy* means providing support when the patient is encountering difficulty, is burdened by stress, or is vulnerable in dealing with reality. It is often short-term or time-limited, helping the patient through a period of crisis. It is one of the basic forms of psychotherapy, which seems to imply that it should be universally applicable. However, it becomes clear on careful examination that *support* must imply an understanding of how to provide such support, in what manner or to what extent, so that it is culturally relevant or appropriate. Therefore, even simple supportive psychotherapy would be subject to cultural modification and proper adjustment.

To begin with, the therapist needs to carefully assess the patient's understanding of psychotherapy in general and his or her expectation of the brief, supportive therapy that is to be carried out. On this basis, it is hoped that the therapist can predict the possible patterns of the patient's adherence to therapy.

In any mode of psychotherapy, the patient-therapist relationship is of paramount importance. This is true in supportive therapy, even though it may be brief. It is well known that the therapist-patient relationship is influenced by various individual factors—including personality, gender, and psychopathology—but it is definitely molded by sociocultural factors. A culturally competent therapist needs to carefully examine the proper therapist-patient relationship in terms of the roles to be played and the level and nature of intimacy to be maintained throughout the therapy. These issues can include physical contact between them and the manner in which support is given in accordance with etiquette (see "Case 1: Using Cultural Differences to Advantage" in this chapter). An area of particular concern involves the gender and age of the therapist and the patient. Relating to patients of different ages and genders should be examined within a cultural context. It is important to establish and maintain a therapeutic alliance that is not only therapeutic but also socioculturally appropriate. A therapist should not ignore the impact of the therapist on the patient through the therapeutic relationship, even if therapy is only for a short period of time. In psychotherapy, even supportive therapy, the therapist will encourage the patient to explore personal life and examine private matters that the patient may never have revealed even to a spouse or other family members—as may be true especially in a society where open communication and revealing one's feelings are not the norm. The psychiatric experience will be a very intimate and unusual one for the patient. It may result in an unexpected transference that needs careful management (see "Case 1: Using Cultural Differences to Advantage" below). Ethnic or cultural transference may occur even in the process of supportive therapy.

When psychopharmacological therapy is to be combined with psychotherapy, it is important for the therapist to know that there are ethnic and racial differences in psychopharmacological responses and that prescribing medication and taking medication often have multiple psychological and sociocultural implications and impacts (see Chapter 10, Culture and Drug Therapy).

The concept and expectation of therapy should be checked out initially and clarified continually to avoid any misunderstandings or misleading expectations. The range and nature of support need to be evaluated against cultural understanding so that the meaning and purpose of therapy will be clear and relevant. The matters of payment and the giving and receiving of gifts should be clarified carefully throughout the course of treatment, because they have different meanings in different cultures. The therapist needs to recognize and use maximally the strengths of the patient and the sources of support from the family, as well as the sociomedical system and cultural environment, to facilitate the patient's improvement.

Psychoanalytically Oriented Psychotherapy

In analytically oriented psychotherapy, it is necessary to first evaluate the capacity of the patient to engage in and utilize psychodynamic psychotherapy. This evaluation should be based on socioeconomic and cultural factors, in addition to frequently considered factors such as individual personality and psychopathology. The patient's level of understanding of dynamic concepts needs to be evaluated and proper interpretation of unconscious material applied accordingly.

Metaphors and symbolic meanings must always be checked against cultural understanding and beliefs. Symbolism is not universal and is subject to cultural factors. The same symbol might be interpreted differently and even in opposite ways in different cultures. For instance, a dragon is viewed as a symbol of evil in the West, whereas in the East it is viewed as a benevolent figure and a symbol of authority (see "Case 2: Cultural Misinterpretations in Analytical Therapy" in this chapter). A snake is generally considered to be a male symbol in the West, but in Eastern societies such as China it could represent a female (such as a seductive woman in a fairy tale). Therefore, it is important that the basic rules of psychoanalysis be applied: it is necessary to understand how a symbol is interpreted by the patient (according to his or her individual and cultural interpretation), but not by the therapist (based on his or her own cultural interpretation) or according to a book.

The therapeutic maneuver of uncovering versus suppression of unconscious affect, drive, or conflict deserves careful consideration and proper choice, depending on the patient's cultural background and cultural definitions of *healthy* and *mature*. In some societies it is considered healthy to spill out deep feelings, whereas in others it is viewed as mature to suppress internal desires.

The interpretation of personal transference deserves careful consideration that takes into account how the therapist-patient relationship is viewed and the cultural expectations of that professional relationship. In addition to *personal* transference and countertransference, there is a need to pay attention to and to manage the possible additional dimensions of *ethnic and cultural* transference and countertransference.

Cognitive Psychotherapy

In cognitive therapy, the basic therapeutic focus is on cognition, with the idea that if the patient could remove distorted or dysfunctional thought and rebuild a healthy, correct cognition, his or her emotions and behavior would be improved. However, from a cultural perspective, the therapist needs to understand that automatic thought and cognitive distortion or dysfunctional behavior need careful evaluation and clarification based on various factors, including sociocultural concepts, definitions, and judgments. In other words, *healthy, unhealthy, functional,* and *dysfunctional* are culturally influenced judgments, and these judgments determine the strategies in cognitive therapy. Even the question of what is mature and what is functional thought needs philosophical examination and consideration. For instance, the philosophical views of "accepting everything as it is" and not "trying to change or remove it," which are rooted in Eastern Daoistic (or Taoistic) views, are very much utilized in the Morita therapy that developed in Japan at the turn of the twentieth century and in the Daoistic cognitive therapy that has emerged recently in China. However, such cognitive views may not be accepted in the West as healthy or functional ways of viewing things, or utilized as the focus for cognitive therapy. In other words, they are heavily subject to cultural judgment.

Behavioral Therapy

In carrying out behavioral therapy, the therapist needs to provide a careful initial explanation and orientation of the therapeutic program because many patients are unfamiliar with programmed therapeutic procedures and the practice of the therapy, which involves providing punishments or rewards to enforce learning and behavior change. The therapist needs to clarify the sociocultural implications of positive and negative reinforcement utilized for behavioral change. In other words, the cultural implications of the rewards and punishments involved in learning need cultural clarification to avoid any misunderstandings.

Marital Therapy

In marital therapy, the therapist usually works on several different areas, including the partners' expectations of and commitment to marriage, the division of roles between husband and wife, ways of rearing children, relationships with families of origin, communication and sharing between partners, and methods of coping when problems arise. Obviously, all of these issues are subject to cultural factors. Therefore, there is a great need for cultural consideration in marital therapy. In practice, the marital therapist needs to pay attention to the culturally defined roles of man and woman, husband and wife, and father and mother. These roles vary greatly in different cultural groups. They may become the cause of problems in intercultural marriages and the focus of subsequent marital therapy (see "Case 3: Couple Therapy for a Filipino American Wife Who Attempted Suicide" in this chapter).

Acceptable, effective ways of dealing with marital problems vary from culture to culture. For instance, openly acknowledging and facing problems and actively—even aggressively—trying to resolve them are coping patterns favored in some cultures, whereas passively enduring and concealing problems to maintain harmony may be considered a virtue in other cultures. It is the therapist's job to check with the couple he or she is treating to learn the nature and direction of their cultural coping patterns. The goals and outcomes of therapy need to be clarified with the couple from the beginning and throughout the course of treatment.

Family Therapy

In family therapy, the therapist needs to be familiar with cultural variations of family systems, structures, and interactional patterns, including family roles, communication, and value systems (Tseng and Hsu 1991). As in marital therapy, the therapist also needs to know how to select culturally suitable intervention techniques, so that culturally relevant family therapies can be applied in families with different cultural backgrounds. For instance, to what extent should the therapist encourage the younger generation to express its views and opinions to the parent generation? For people living in a relatively conservative society that emphasizes the hierarchy between family members, it would be a mistake to encourage the youngsters to openly and publicly criticize their parents during a session. Even though in a society in which open communication is valued it would be considered therapeutic to encourage family members to express their opinions and feelings and to communicate openly, it would still be perceived as insulting and impolite behavior by traditional parents and might produce undesirable results, if not disaster (see "Case 4: Teenage Sons Encouraged to Criticize Their Father" in this chapter). What constitutes a normal, healthy family is subject to cultural variation. This always needs to be considered when conducting family therapy with families of different cultural backgrounds.

Group Therapy

Group therapy involves a group of members in therapeutic activities. Activities include group formation, interaction, and processes. In addition to the basic factors relating to group composition—including age, gender, personality, and the psychopathology of the members—the group transactions will obviously be influenced by the ethnic and cultural backgrounds of the members and the therapist.

For instance, a patient who comes from a Mexican tradition of close-mouthedness and not opening up to others (*no te rajes*) will affect the process of communication and expression of feelings in group situations (Martinez 1977). Clinicians who work with Spanish-speaking groups may find that there is a built-in formality in interpersonal relations among the members that is reflected in their language usage. This greater formality can make it difficult for group members to relate to one another candidly as equals and can inhibit the expression of negative feelings toward the therapist. Based on group therapy experiences with Chinese clients in Canada, Chen (1995) noted that the Chinese patients tended to expect the therapist to maintain the image of an authority figure with expertise, to educate the group members, and to provide structure for the group process. Chen also noted that it was preferable for the therapist to define rules and boundaries for the members to follow.

These examples indicate that the behavior of group members is greatly influenced by their cultural backgrounds in the areas of communication style, relational patterns, and interaction with the therapist, all of which in turn affect the process of group therapy. In contrast to individual psychotherapy, which focuses mainly on the psychopathology of an individual, interpersonal psychotherapy deals primarily with problems related to interpersonal issues; thus there is more of a need to consider and understand the impact of culture on interactional human behavior.

When a group's membership is multiethnic, the situation becomes much more complicated from a cultural perspective, and there is a great need for attention to several issues, such as encouraging the explanation and exploration of ethnically derived values to help the members understand the interpersonal behavior that results from these values, helping the members observe and understand culture-rooted nonverbal and symbolic forms of communication, exploring the dynamics underlying the cultural transferences arising from group members, examining cultural transferences occurring within the therapist(s), and helping the members examine their ethnic or racial prejudices in a safe environment that can contain the strong affects that arise (Matsukawa 2001).

Case Vignettes With Discussion

Case 1: Using Cultural Differences to Advantage

Mrs. Stoltz, a middle-aged European American patient, was treated for depression with supportive therapy by a Chinese resident therapist. When Mrs. Stoltz was crying, expressing her feelings of sorrow, the young resident, without thinking, patted the patient's shoulder to comfort her. During the supervision session, the resident described this therapeutic encounter to the supervisor, who pointed out to the resident therapist that such physical contact was not professionally appropriate for that patient, even though it may have been individually and culturally acceptable to the therapist.

The therapist was eager to help this depressed and incapacitated patient to find external support in her own environment. However, the therapist himself was new to the society and was not knowledgeable of the social support systems that were available to the patient. Therefore, the therapist had to consult a social worker to explore the support systems in the local community, including where to seek financial help and how to establish a social network.

However, in the treatment session the therapist was able to quote many Chinese proverbs to comfort the patient and encourage her to regain hope. For instance, the therapist would mention the old Chinese saying, "If you have a green mountain in your back yard, you would not worry all of your life that there would be no wood for cooking," implying that if you are healthy, you have no problem coping with difficulties in life. The therapist also told the patient the story of Mr. Sai and his horse. In this story an old man, Mr. Sai, lost his horse but later acquired a wild horse; his son injured his leg by riding the wild horse, but then he was waived from being drafted during the war and did not lose his life as other young men from his village did. The story implies that situations in life can change unpredictably from misfortune to good fortune, so there is no need to feel desperate when misfortune occurs. Mrs. Stoltz was very much impressed and encouraged by these Eastern sayings.

The therapy went on smoothly without further complications for several months, providing the patient with emotional support and help with life adjustment. Not having detected anything unusual, the therapist was surprised at the last session when Mrs. Stoltz appeared wearing a yellow dress and yellow stockings, with her hair dyed black, and with a book of Confucius in her hands. Mrs. Stoltz talked about how much she benefited from the therapy and how she would miss the therapist after termination of the time-limited therapy. She said that she would remember what the therapist had wisely advised her in the past and would consult the Confucius book whenever she had concerns. Mrs. Stoltz developed an intense identification with the therapist whom she was losing, manifesting this identification at the ethnic level.

Case 2: Cultural Misinterpretations in Analytical Therapy

Mr. Lee, an Asian patient, was treated by a Western psychoanalyst. In the early stages of therapy, Mr. Lee, following his culturally customary practice, brought a gift to the therapist to indicate his respect and appreciation of the therapist. It was a bamboo plate with a picture of a dragon on it. The therapist, according to his analytical training, not only refused to accept the gift from the patient (to maintain neutrality with the patient) but was also very much puzzled by the symbolic meaning of the dragon picture on the gift. He was concerned as to why Mr. Lee would give him a gift with such a terrifying figure on it. In response to the therapist's inquiry, Mr. Lee explained that a dragon is considered a rain god who will bring needed rain to the land. The dragon represents a benevolent, protective authority figure. Despite the patient's explanation, the analyst remained concerned until he consulted a cultural psychiatrist, who assured him that Mr. Lee's explanation was culturally correct. The cultural psychiatrist also advised the analyst that it would be a good idea to accept Mr. Lee's gift without doubting the motivation or intent of such behavior. The gift should be regarded as a gesture of appreciation to the therapist, representing the hope that the therapist would take good care of him as a patient.

As therapy progressed, the therapist learned that as a boy, Mr. Lee slept with his parents until he was 8 years old. He became sick easily as a small child, and his mother wanted to make sure Mr. Lee was well covered by the quilt in the evening so that he did not catch cold. The therapist was impressed by this information about Mr. Lee's early childhood and interpreted it to mean that the patient was dependent on and over-attached to his mother. The patient tried very hard to explain that all of his peer friends slept with their parents until they were in grade school, but the therapist took it that the patient was making an excuse. With some doubt, the therapist again consulted the cultural psychiatrist, who confirmed that in many parts of Asia it was not unusual for young children to sleep with their parents for many years, particularly if the family did not have an extra bedroom for the children to sleep in.

After the treatment went on for a while, the therapist began to formulate the theory that Mr. Lee's main problems related to an Oedipus complex. The patient was very close to and dependent on his mother and was distant from and fearful of his father. Without too much hesitation, the therapist made the interpretation that Mr. Lee had the unconscious desire to get rid of his father and to possess his mother. These comments particularly disturbed Mr. Lee. His response to the therapist's interpretation was that it was absurd. Mr. Lee explained that in a society that emphasizes filial piety, every son is very close to his mother, and nothing is unusual about this. Clearly, the therapist made a mistake by making this interpretation either prematurely or incorrectly. Mr. Lee never came back for the following session, giving up the treatment.

Case 3: Couple Therapy for a Filipino American Wife Who Attempted Suicide

Marital therapy was arranged for Mr. and Mrs. Simmons after Mrs. Simmons attempted suicide. She had migrated from the Philippines to Hawaii several years before and had married a Caucasian man. Mr. and Mrs. Simmons described their relationship as having started with love at first sight. They married soon after they met. His parents did not attend the wedding because they did not approve of his intermarriage.

Her family did not attend either, because it was too expensive for them to come from the Philippines. Despite this, Mr. and Mrs. Simmons claimed that they were happily married and having a satisfactory life.

After Mrs. Simmons became pregnant, her husband invited his parents to visit them in Hawaii. He thought that it would be a good time for his parents to meet his wife and become close as a family. However, things did not go as planned. Mrs. Simmons had severe morning sickness and was very much annoyed that her husband spent more time with his parents than with her. Despite her warnings, Mr. Simmons continued to spend considerable time showing his parents around, hoping that they would enjoy their visit. With his mother now physically disabled, Mr. Simmons thought that it might be his last chance to be close to her and be nice to her. Mrs. Simmons became hysterical, overdosed, and was sent to the emergency room.

The history revealed that this was not the first time Mrs. Simmons had experienced emotional turmoil. Before the parents' visit, Mr. Simmons's sister had come to visit. Mrs. Simmons had a serious quarrel with her husband when he prepared the bed for his sister rather than let his wife, as hostess, do it. Furthermore, it upset Mrs. Simmons very much when the three of them went out in the car. The husband drove the car as usual, but asked his sister to sit next to him, letting his wife sit in the back seat. Mrs. Simmons assumed that her husband cared more for his sister than he did for his own wife. She cried and caused a scene at home, and her sister-in-law left the uncomfortable situation.

From a clinical point of view, multiple factors contributed to the problems. The interracial marriage might have contributed indirectly; however, personality and interpersonal relationship patterns between them played an important part.

In therapy, this couple was encouraged to discuss, communicate, and explain their behaviors to each other. With regard to Mr. Simmons letting his sister sit in the front seat next him, with help from the therapist Mr. Simmons explained that because it was the first time his sister had come to this new place, he thought that letting her sit in the front seat would allow her to sightsee better. Mrs. Simmons accused him of not taking the time to explain his intentions, letting her feel that she was being treated as a "second citizen" to her sister-in-law. As for the situation relating to his parents' visit, he explained that he hoped by being nice to his parents and making them happy, they would become nicer to his wife in return. But Mrs. Simmons pointed out that she was experiencing morning sickness at that time and badly needed her husband's attention and care. Mrs. Simmons, not having her own parents nearby (they were far away in the Philippines), felt terribly lonely and felt she was being deserted by her husband.

Mr. Simmons did not have many complaints about his wife, except that she would frequently send money to her parents, siblings, and even more distant relatives in the Philippines. He felt that, after marriage, a husband and wife should keep some distance from the family of origin. He certainly did not want to have responsibility for financially supporting his in-laws.

The therapist explained, using simple words, that the boundaries among self, surrounding persons, and particularly families of origin vary in different cultures. Even though a person is married, in a family-oriented society such as the Philippines there is a continuous bond between self and family, and this includes financial obligation; whereas in individual-oriented societies such as the United States the bond will diminish after marriage in favor of the formation of a new family. This was one cultural issue that Mr. and Mrs. Simmons needed to work out between them.

The therapist pointed out to them that from the information presented to him, he had the impression that, as husband and wife, they had affection between them and were getting along well most of the time, except in their relations with their families of origin and at the times when their family members visited them. These were usually critical times that stirred up the need for readjustment of the emotional ties to their families of origin and within their own newly formed family. The therapist indicated that there was a need for the new couple to learn how to adjust the roles of husband and wife in different circumstances depending on their own individual tastes and choices as well as the values and customs they were raised with. The therapist encouraged them to work out the different views that they might have by engaging in more direct communication and explanation, searching for solutions for themselves, both the individual and the cultural level.

The couple responded to the therapy rather favorably by learning how to communicate and negotiate between them more than before. They became especially happy after their baby was born. No major problems were detected even several years later.

Case 4: Teenage Sons Encouraged to Criticize Their Father

Mr. and Mrs. Pak sought treatment at a family clinic. They brought their three sons, David, age 15 years; John, 13; and Bobby, 8. Both David and John were taller and appeared stronger than their father. Mr. Pak, a Korean American, was very strict in his manner of disciplining his children. He expected them to do their chores at home and follow his orders without complaint. Mrs. Pak, a European American, was more liberal and was emotionally close to her children. She was inclined to allow them to make decisions for themselves, thinking it would encourage their maturation.

In recent months, a constant tension had developed between Mr. Pak and his two older sons. For instance, one night John failed to take out the garbage immediately after being told to do so by Mr. Pak. Mr. Pak ended up shouting at John. John talked back to his father, enraging Mr. Pak. A few days before the family session, Mr. Pak asked David to pick up a stick that had been left in the yard, and David did not do it immediately. Mr. Pak then picked up the stick and threatened to hit David, while David, larger and stronger than his father, put up his fists and threatened to fight back. This conflict between her husband and her teenage sons made Mrs. Pak fearful that a dangerous physical fight might erupt among them. She threatened to leave the family unless they all agreed to see a family therapist.

During the family session, Mr. Pak revealed that when he was growing up in Korea his own father had been very strict. Mr. Pak had learned to respectfully follow any command given by his parents, and he certainly would never have talked back to them. Based on the way he was raised, Mr. Pak could not tolerate his own children's behavior. He stated his belief that youngsters nowadays were spoiled and needed more discipline. Mrs. Pak reported that during her upbringing in her Caucasian family there had seldom been loud arguments, and there was certainly no physical discipline. She expressed the belief that times had changed and that her husband should understand that children grow up differently now and he must learn to relate to the children based on their needs.

The therapist identified more with Mrs. Pak's position. The therapist chose to promote communication among the family members, hoping that each would come to understand how the other feels, which would improve their relationship. The two sons, David and John, were encouraged by the therapist to speak up, explaining how they felt about their father's behavior. David described how his father treated him as if he was still a small child, ordering him around, forgetting that he had grown up and was already in high school. The therapist praised David for being able to express his opinions in front of everyone.

Following this, John in turn complained that his father was too fussy, getting upset if everything was not done exactly his own way. John started to imitate how his father would nag and scold the children. As John was doing so, the youngest son, Bobby, sitting next to Mr. Pak, giggled. Hearing this, Mr. Pak turned to Bobby and slapped his face before the therapist had time to intervene. Bobby cried and ran to his mother. Embarrassed, Mr. Pak announced that there was no good in having such family sessions, and he refused to return to therapy.

In retrospect, the therapist came to realize that the attempts to promote communication had led to the criticism of Mr. Pak, which shamed him in front of his family and also a stranger (the therapist), thus causing him to lose face. His sons were disrespecting him, and Bobby's laughter was more than he could bear. Even though, in principle, a goal of family therapy is to facilitate communication and mutual understanding among family members, the therapist failed to recognize that such communication requires a culturally appropriate structure, and the therapist needed to devise a communication system that could bridge the two cultural styles.

Clinical Suggestions for Culturally Competent Psychotherapy

1. *Be aware of cultural impact beyond general factors.* The competent psychotherapist needs to be aware of factors that will influence the process and outcome of psychotherapy. These include the patient's

personality and life experience and the psychopathology that the patient is experiencing. Beyond that, the therapist needs to know the cultural factors that may influence the content and also the process of psychological treatment. These are described more specifically later in this section.

2. *Establish and maintain a culturally adjusted therapist-patient relationship.* The therapist-patient relationship is a core issue in psychotherapy. It involves social boundaries, physical distance, and an authority-subordinate relationship. All these factors are variable within limits. Establishing and maintaining these limits requires adjustment according to the cultures of the therapist and the patient, not just the specific type of psychotherapy. This adjustment should be integrated with what is desirable from a therapeutic point of view.

3. *Foster culturally relevant communication.* Psychotherapy is carried out mainly in the form of communication between the therapist and the patient. However, communication is determined by the language, the pattern of communication, and the purpose of communication. It is deeply influenced by levels of intelligence, cognitive styles, social customs, and cultural patterns of communication. Which subjects to explore, to what extent, with what objective, and how much the patient can accept and tolerate the area of exploration are all factors that need to be considered. More specifically, to what extent it can be therapeutic to explore subconscious material, to reveal underlying desires, or to interpret emotional conflict depends on cultural factors in addition to other general factors.

4. *Develop culture-oriented psychodynamic understanding.* Formulating an explanation for the patient's symptomatic behaviors, thoughts, and feelings allows development of a specific therapeutic strategy. Incorporating cultural issues into the formulation requires more than just cultural sensitivity. The degree of cultural knowledge and insight needed to capture a truly meaningful understanding for therapy may extend beyond the knowledge and ability of the therapist and might require consultation with cultural experts.

5. *Select a culturally suitable mode of psychotherapy.* Most clinicians believe that the mode of psychotherapy that should be used depends on the specific psychopathology of the patient. In addition, a patient's ethnic and cultural background helps determine the suitability of a given mode of psychotherapy. The degree to which the patient is familiar with the nature and process of therapy and is comfortable with a given kind of approach influences his or her readiness to benefit from a particular type of therapy. Little is known about the varying responses of different cultural groups to modes of

therapy. Often trial and error are necessary rather than following specific rules.

6. *Utilize culturally sanctioned coping mechanisms.* The goal of psychotherapy is to help patients deal with their problems. Psychotherapy enhances patients' coping mechanisms or helps them learn new ways to prevent or manage problems. Some coping mechanisms are more familiar to the patient, whereas others that are less utilized by the patient may be more effective. Some coping mechanisms are also more likely to be sanctioned by society and culture. Techniques to enhance such culturally sanctioned coping patterns are a consideration for the therapist and the patient to explore and discuss, and to apply if they are judged to be useful, therapeutic, and effective.

7. *Adjust definitions of health and maturity to take cultural judgments into account.* The goal of psychotherapy is to help the patient become more healthy and mature. However, *healthy* and *mature* are not only defined professionally but are subject to social and cultural judgment. If the goals of therapy are culturally consonant and desirable to the patient, they are more likely to be achieved.

8. *Be aware of the implications of psychotherapy's effect on culture.* A competent therapist should comprehend the implications of psychotherapy on culture. Psychotherapy can influence culturally rooted values, beliefs, and behaviors. It can affirm central cultural values, provide culturally permitted channels for fulfillment of wishes or desires, reinforce culturally sanctioned coping patterns, permit cultural "time out," explore alternative cultural approaches to resolving problems, and foster the elaboration and incorporation of new cultural systems (Tseng and Hsu 1979).

The nature of psychotherapy can be regarded as the interaction between two value systems: that of the patient and that of the therapist. Through the process of therapy, a patient is exposed to the therapist's way of viewing things, which is supposedly more healthy and functional than the patient's way. After the process of exchange and incorporation, the patient absorbs this healthier value system to some extent. Therefore, in a microscopic way, certain aspects of an acculturation process take place through the process of psychotherapy. Thus, beyond considerations of technical, theoretical, and philosophical modifications—or cultural adjustments to suit the ethnic and cultural background of the patient—a self-examination by the therapist of his or her own cultural background and value system is equally important, because it can form the basis for the way the therapist or the patient is influenced in the process of psychotherapy.

References

Chen CP: Group counseling in a different cultural context: several primary issues in dealing with Chinese clients. Group 19:45–55, 1995

Frank JD: Persuasion and Healing: A Comparative Study of Psychotherapy. New York, Schocken Books, 1961

Martinez C: Group process and the Chicano: clinical issues. Int J Group Psychother 27:225–231, 1977

Matsukawa LA: Group therapy with multiethnic members, in Culture and Psychotherapy: A Guide to Clinical Practice. Edited by Tseng WS, Streltzer J. Washington, DC, American Psychiatric Press, 2001, pp 243–261

Pedersen PB, Draguns JG, Lonner WJ, et al: Counseling Across Cultures, 4th Edition. Thousand Oaks, CA, Sage, 1996

Prince R: Variations in psychotherapy procedures, in Handbook of Cross-Cultural Psychology: Psychopathology, Vol 6. Edited by Triandis HC, Draguns JG. Boston, MA, Allyn & Bacon, 1980, pp 291–349

Torrey EF: Witchdoctor and Psychiatrist: The Common Roots of Psychotherapy and Its Future. New York, Harper & Row, 1986

Tseng WS: Psychotherapy for the Chinese: cultural adjustment, in Psychotherapy for the Chinese, Vol II. Edited by Cheng LYC, Baxter H, Cheung FMC. Hong Kong, Chinese University of Hong Kong, 1995, pp 1–22

Tseng WS: Culture and psychotherapy: review and practical guidance. Transcult Psychiatry 36:131–179, 1999

Tseng WS: Handbook of Cultural Psychiatry. San Diego, CA, Academic Press, 2001

Tseng WS: Clinician's Guide to Cultural Psychiatry. San Diego, CA, Academic Press, 2003

Tseng WS, Hsu J: Culture and psychotherapy, in Perspectives on Cross-Cultural Psychology. Edited by Marsella AJ, Tharp RG, Ciborowski TJ. New York, Academic Press, 1979, pp 333–345

Tseng WS, Hsu J: Culture and Family: Problems and Therapy. New York, Haworth, 1991

Tseng WS, Streltzer J (eds): Culture and Psychotherapy: A Guide for Clinical Practice. Washington, DC, American Psychiatric Press, 2001

Wohl J: Integration of cultural awareness into psychotherapy. Am J Psychother 43:343–355, 1989

Index